James Le Fanu has combined a career as a General Practitioner in South London with writing about medicine and science for the *Sunday* and *Daily Telegraph*. He has also contributed articles and reviews to *The Times*, *Spectator*, *New Statesman*, *Literary Review*, *British Medical Journal* and *Journal of The Royal Society of Medicine*. His much acclaimed *The Rise and Fall of Modern Medicine* won the *Los Angeles Times* book prize in 2001. His most recent book, *Why Us?*, was published jointly by HarperCollins in the UK and Random House in the US in 2009. He was elected a Fellow of the Royal College of Physicians in 2014.

Also by this author

The Rise and Fall of Modern Medicine

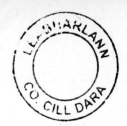

Too Many Pills

How Too Much Medicine is Endangering Our Health and What We Can Do About It

JAMES LE FANU

Little, Brown

LITTLE, BROWN

First published in Great Britain by Little, Brown in 2018

5 7 9 10 8 6

A CIP catalogue record for this book
is available from the British Library.

ISBN 978-1-4087-0977-1

Typeset in Caslon by M Rules
Printed and bound in Great Britain by
Clays Ltd, Elcograf S.p.A.

Papers used by Little, Brown are from well-managed forests
and other responsible sources.

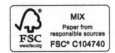

Little, Brown
An imprint of
Little, Brown Book Group
Carmelite House
50 Victoria Embankment
London EC4Y 0DZ

An Hachette UK Company
www.hachette.co.uk

www.littlebrown.co.uk

To my parents
in memoriam

Disclaimer

The information in this book is not intended to replace or conflict with the advice given to you by your GP or other health professionals. All matters regarding your health including any medication that you take should be discussed with your GP. The author and publisher disclaim any liability directly or indirectly from the use of the material in this book by any person.

The physician must have two special objects in view ... namely to do good and do no harm

Hippocrates: *Epidemics*, Book 1

Contents

List of Figures and Tables

List of Figures and Tables

Introduction

'Tis impossible to separate the chance of good
from the risk of ill

David Hume

In just fifteen years the number of prescriptions issued by family doctors in Britain has increased three-fold. Everyone agrees this is too many – a regular topic of conversation down the pub, on the golf course and the bowling green. Some are apprehensive about even visiting the surgery lest they be burdened with taking yet more drugs: 'Quite a number of people I know are fearful of seeing their family doctors because of this.' Dutiful children visiting their parents or elderly relatives are aghast at the six, or eight, or ten different types of pill cluttering the bathroom cabinet.

Doctors themselves certainly recognise the problem, with nine out of ten GPs in a straw poll acknowledging that they prescribe 'too many pills'. The *British Medical Journal*, among others, has published numerous articles on the subject and along with several academic institutions has sponsored five international conferences – in Oxford, Washington, Barcelona, Quebec and Copenhagen – on the theme 'Rolling back the harms of too much medicine'. Popular campaigns – 'Choosing wisely' in the United States, 'Slow medicine' in Italy – seek to mitigate the consequences.

'The consequences' are, of course, the nub of the matter. For, as the Scottish philosopher David Hume observed, ''Tis impossible to separate the chance of good from the risk of ill.' There is no drug intended to do good that does not cause harm in some. And the more that are taken, the greater the chances. Over the past ten years, thousands of readers of my weekly medical column have written to tell of the misery of the muscular aches and pains, lethargy, insomnia, impaired concentration, gut disturbances and general decrepitude caused by their drugs – and their almost miraculous recovery on discontinuing them. The adverse consequences of 'polypharmacy' (literally, many pills) are vastly greater than is commonly appreciated, being responsible for a remarkable 75 per cent increase in recent years in the numbers requiring emergency hospital admission for adverse drug reactions. And polypharmacy can also be fatal, almost certainly a contributory factor to the recently observed decline in life expectancy – six hundred more people dying every week in 2015 compared to previous years.

So how did this situation arise? The origins of polypharmacy can be traced back to two very radical ideas. More than forty years ago, Henry Gadsden, the brilliant chairman of (at the time) the world's largest and most innovative drug company, Merck, proposed that the future prosperity of the pharmaceutical industry would require expanding the market for its products beyond merely treating the ill to include the healthy as well. Ideally, he would like to 'sell to everyone'. Ten years later a prominent British epidemiologist, Professor Geoffrey Rose,

2

provided, if unintentionally, the rationale by which Gadsden's rather disturbing vision might be realised. It is not just individuals who are ill, argued Rose; rather 'the population is sick'. The blood pressure, cholesterol and glucose levels in the population are on average 'too high' and there is more to be gained by lowering these measurements in millions of people than by focusing on the relatively few in whom they are markedly elevated. This is, admittedly, a difficult concept to comprehend (it will become clear enough), but the notion of the 'population approach' – as it is known – of treating the many remains a central principle of medical thinking, to be exploited by the pharmaceutical industry to its immensely profitable advantage over several decades.

The third crucial element, closing the circle as it were, of too much medicine is more recent. In 2004, the long-standing contractual arrangements by which family doctors are remunerated were overturned in favour of 'payment by performance', financially incentivised to maximise the number of their patients being treated for a list of conditions. The synergy of these three 'players' in promoting polypharmacy, albeit for very different reasons, is now deeply entrenched, institutionalised within current medical practice.

There is thus an understandable reluctance to acknowledge its consequences. The Norwegians aptly describe the situation as 'getting one's foot stuck in the piano', where the discordant noise caused by trying to disentangle it from the strings only draws attention to the gravity of the problems involved.

Hence, for ordinary people, the only way out of this grievous situation is to take the initiative by becoming better acquainted with the current enthusiasm for mass medication and asking more searching questions about the benefits and risks of the drugs they are taking. 'Hang on a minute,' some might say. 'Are you seriously suggesting that, having read your book, I should tell my doctor I no longer wish to take my pills? That is going to be very unpopular, not to say irresponsible, and I wouldn't be surprised if the General Medical Council were to strike you off the register for "bringing the profession into disrepute".'

I take the point. But my interpretation of the rise of poly-pharmacy and its consequences is scarcely unique, reflecting, as mentioned above, the views of many. This book does, however, fill an important gap. It is time to move beyond complaining that doctors now prescribe too many pills to doing something about it. This 'popular' account seeks to provide in a comprehensible way, and for the first time, the relevant evidence by which people can make their own reasoned judgement about widely prescribed medicines – and why it is now generally accepted that two-thirds (or more) of those taking several types of drug gain no benefit from doing so.

Still, I am very aware of a nagging credibility gap – can this possibly be true? Medicine is, after all, a highly respected science-based profession guided by well-defined ethical values that could scarcely tolerate the folly of polypharmacy and the drive to expand ever further the number of the medicalised.

There is, however, an historical precedent for the events described in this book in the publication just over fifty years ago in 1967 by Maurice Pappworth of *Human Guinea Pigs*, an anthology of the cruel, dangerous and often purposeless experiments carried out in leading academic centres on infants, pregnant women, the mentally ill, the old and dying. Thus, in one typical experiment the participants were required to exercise on a standing bicycle with a tight mask fitted over the face while a thin catheter inserted through a large-bore needle in the arm monitored pressure within the heart. Not a pleasant experience for anyone, but, Pappworth pointed out, all the subjects were seriously ill, suffering from cancer, anaemia or various forms of lung disease. The roll call of those responsible for the experiments (and he mentions 126 by name) included most of the eminent and distinguished physicians of his time. They were scandalised, and he inevitably paid a high price, being ostracised by the medical establishment till almost the end of his career.

The significance of this precedent is two-fold. First, doctors may not be aware of the extent of the miseries inflicted by polypharmacy and indeed of the flawed reasoning and sophistry with which it has been so vigorously promoted. Next, Pappworth, in the introduction to *Human Guinea Pigs*, emphasises in bold his central concern, which is highly relevant to what follows. It reads:

> **'In the great majority of articles giving accounts of these experiments, the authors do not mention whether consent was obtained. Therefore, in any particular example cited, unless definitely stated to the contrary, we must not assume that valid consent was given.'**

Similarly, any decision to initiate treatment that involves, as in many cases, taking a drug indefinitely, requires first obtaining the patient's truly informed consent – a proper understanding of the benefits (which may well be very small) and potential adverse effects. This does not happen. My hope in writing this book is that it will allow readers to have that discussion with their doctors. In the following chapter I shall elaborate on this Introduction as a prelude to examining in some detail the five main 'pillars' of polypharmacy.

Chapter 1

Too Much Medicine

Over the past sixty years, medicine has metamorphosed from a modest pursuit of limited effectiveness into a massive global phenomenon employing millions and costing trillions. Now, in the vast shiny palace the modern hospital has become, the previously unimaginable goals of transplanting organs and curing childhood cancer have become unexceptional while every year tens of thousands previously doomed to blindness from cataracts or to immobility from crippling arthritis have their sight and mobility restored. Medicine has become the most visible symbol of the fulfilment of the promise that scientific progress would vanquish the twin perils of ignorance and disease to the benefit of all.

And yet the more powerful and prestigious medicine has become, the greater the impetus to extend its influence yet further, resulting in the progressive 'medicalisation' of people's lives to no good purpose. This takes many forms: unnecessary tests, the over-treatment of minor symptoms, the inappropriate use of the life-sustaining technologies of the intensive care unit, a constant stream of – often contradictory – warnings about trivial or non-existent threats to health in people's everyday lives, and unreasonable claims as to what the current state of medical research can reasonably be expected to achieve.

The most serious form of that medicalisation, by far, is 'too many pills' – the mass prescribing of drugs, imposing a serious burden on people's lives while (if paradoxically) posing a substantial threat to their health and wellbeing. In the very recent past the number of prescriptions issued by family doctors in Britain has increased three-fold – so it is now not unusual for those in their seventies and beyond to be taking a cocktail of numerous different drugs, with twice as many taking more than five, three times as many ten or more.

The several explanations for this dramatic 'rise in polypharmacy' include most obviously the reality that, as ever more people live ever longer, they become vulnerable to the inevitable 'chronic diseases of ageing', which can be mitigated, if not vanquished, by painkillers, anti-inflammatory drugs, acid suppressants, heart and water pills, and so on. Then it could be an indication of doctors' greater thoroughness in diagnosing and treating ailments that may previously have been overlooked. The discovery of novel drugs such as Viagra extends the range of treatable conditions yet further, while the development of medicines better tolerated than those they replace (such as the antidepressant Prozac) lowers the bar for initiating treatment – accounting, at least in part, for the additional two million people who take them compared to twenty years ago. It may be, too, that the public have become more demanding of their doctors, insisting for example on being prescribed antibiotics for relatively minor coughs, colds and sore throats that might be expected to improve of their own accord. This is certainly a common perception but, perhaps surprisingly, during this period prescriptions for antibiotics have remained virtually static at just over three million a year.

These several possibilities are eclipsed by the main driving force behind the rise of polypharmacy, the extension of the sound principle of treating those with markedly raised blood pressure, sugar or cholesterol levels – in anticipation of reducing their risk of heart attack, stroke or the complications of diabetes – to the millions in whom these parameters are only modestly elevated, if at all. This widening of the scope of those deemed eligible for treatment is reflected in the truly awesome seven-fold increase in the numbers of prescriptions for blood pressure-lowering medications, a five-fold rise in diabetic drugs and a twenty-fold increase in the cholesterol-lowering statins (see Figure 1.1). Still, the logic behind that dizzying upward spiral in the number of prescriptions is plausible enough. There are very few more useful things a doctor can do than prevent the catastrophe of stroke by prescribing blood pressure-lowering drugs. To be sure, it is the relatively few with severe hypertension who are most likely to benefit, but a fair proportion of strokes occur in those with 'mild' hypertension, who would be similarly advantaged by drugs that can add twenty or more years to a person's life. Ditto cholesterol and blood sugar.

Fair enough. But the common feature of those 'physiological variables' (as they are known) of blood pressure, cholesterol and sugar levels is that they *are* variable. They fluctuate in response to circumstances and over time. The stress and worries of everyday life may, for some, increase the blood pressure, which then returns to normal once they are resolved. Those variables also

Figure 1.1 Too much medicine: The phenomenal rise in the number of prescriptions for the most commonly prescribed classes of drug in the UK 1994–2012

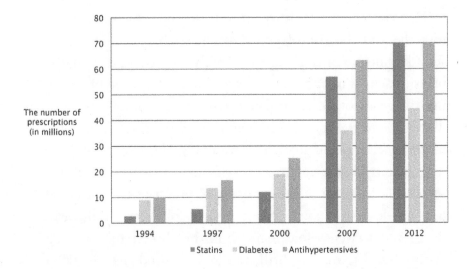

rise with age, so a raised measurement for someone in their thirties becomes 'average' for a person in their seventies. Or again, and very importantly, those variables tend to be higher in the plump than in the thin and will fall back within the normal range by the simple expedient of shedding, by dietary means, a stone or more in weight. The upshot being that, if this variability is not taken into account when diagnosing hypertension, diabetes or 'high cholesterol', then substantial numbers will end up being treated for a condition they do not have.

That aside, the argument for 'mass' medication might seem intuitively undesirable for several common-sense reasons. First, the authoritative advice to millions that, while they may believe themselves to be fit and healthy, one or more of their physiological measurements is 'too high' can induce morbid

10

preoccupations, transforming the 'well' into the 'worried well'. The following scenario, described by a recently retired lawyer, will be familiar to many:

'It is my extreme good fortune to have enjoyed robust good health all my adult life that I put down to a legacy of parental genes, healthy eating, red wine and exercise – and a lifelong aversion to taking any medication.'

At the age of sixty-five he receives a letter from his GP's surgery inviting him to attend for a flu jab:

'At the clinic, the nurse looked at my record and almost scolded me for my absence over all these years. Reluctantly I was persuaded to attend the "well man check-up" where I was duly weighed and measured and gave various samples for testing. And then the triumphant: "Ah ha! Gotcha!" was uttered when my blood pressure was taken and found to be raised. The doctor told me I would hereafter be on a regime of several pills to control my blood pressure for the rest of my life – starting with a low dose of the one on the prescription he was now writing. I was now a patient – eternally dependent upon medication with more to come! There was no comfort reading the side-effects leaflet in the box with my tablets. This did not mention insomnia, but for the first time in my life I suffered from it, worrying about how my life had changed. Ignorance being bliss I had always felt well, but no longer.'

Then, the burden of complex drug regimes is onerous, seriously compromising the quality of people's lives. A man in his late seventies taking half a dozen different drugs writes:

'I have got a book and I note everything down: the time, the drug, and when I've taken it. When you are busy around the house or otherwise engaged you can quite easily forget to take them and sometimes you don't really know whether you have taken them or not. So, I make a point of noting down the drug taken and the time taken and tick it off. So, if I think I missed taking a pill, I take a look and, if I haven't ticked it off, do so.'

Next, while the everyday routine practice of medicine remains much the same as ever, the rise of polypharmacy alters the nature of the 'clinical encounter' away from doctors sympathetically engaging their patients in conversation, diagnosing what is amiss and putting it right, in favour of staring at their computer screens and monitoring the effects of the drugs they have prescribed. One woman writes:

'Whenever visiting the surgery nowadays, I find what I want to discuss is increasingly irrelevant. Rather the doctor takes it upon himself to bully me into letting him measure my blood pressure, have a cholesterol test or generally badger me about "lifestyle issues". I resent this authoritarian attitude. It is as if I am being treated like someone who cannot be trusted to make her own decisions.'

Doctors too resent being required to be continually checking up on those 'physiological variables'.

'The biggest change over the course of my career has been the [necessity] to bring healthy people into the surgery and turn them into patients,' writes Glasgow family doctor Margaret McCartney. 'I am no longer there to make people better, I am there to find out what risk factors they might have or could have, despite their feeling well and having no complaints at all. General practice should be there to deal with people who are in physical or mental pain, or who have noticed a worrying lump or who need their diabetes medication adjusting. Hence the paradox: if you are ill, you may have to be persistent and determined to get help. Yet if you are well, you are at risk of being checked and screened into patient-hood, given preventive medication for something you will never get, or treated for something you haven't got.'

It is, as always, necessary to keep a sense of proportion about all this. Medicine remains a highly successful endeavour whose task, despite the disenchantment of patients and the frustration of Dr McCartney and her colleagues, of relieving the burden of ill health continues as before. This brings us to the fourth and most important common-sense reason for doubting the wisdom of polypharmacy. There is no drug that will not cause side effects in some people. The more drugs taken, the greater the likelihood, through their interaction, of those side effects. The more drugs taken by those in their seventies and over whose ability to tolerate them may be compromised by impaired functioning of the liver or kidney, the greater the likelihood they will experience side effects. When millions of people are taking potent medicines to lower their blood pressure or cholesterol, then the numbers experiencing side effects will run into the hundreds of thousands at least. Here it is necessary to note that the term 'side effect' or, in technical terms, 'adverse drug reaction' (ADR), though widely used in this context, is misleading as it conveys the impression this is a minor or incidental inconvenience compared to the therapeutic benefits the drug confers

But this is not the case. The symptoms of headaches, vertigo, dizziness, nausea, vomiting, muscular aches and pains, etc., are no different in the distress they cause than if they were due to a medical condition. This situation where medical intervention is responsible for causing physical suffering rather than alleviating it is known as 'iatrogenic ('iatro' – medicine, 'genic' – induced) harm'. 'The number of patients seriously injured or killed by drug-induced disease is vast', observes one of the contributors to the hefty *Oxford Textbook of Iatrogenic Diseases*, which runs to one thousand pages each of whose forty chapters is a compendium of the findings of hundreds of investigations into its diverse manifestations. 'The range of illnesses is so wide that no solution to this problem seems likely to emerge.'

The rise of polypharmacy will, by necessity, have increased the burden of iatrogenic illness. For those who are fit and well, this should be easy enough to identify as the reason for the onset of, for example, crippling muscular aches and pains soon after initiating drug treatment, and the appropriate remedial action – discontinuing the medication – will be straightforward. The difficulty arises when those iatrogenic illnesses go unrecognised for what they are because their symptoms are insidious, or are misinterpreted as being due to 'getting on' or wrongly attributed to some other condition – resulting in the prescribing of yet further medication to minimise the symptoms they cause.

My first intimation of the scale of this epidemic of 'hidden' iatrogenic illness was prompted by the response to a short item in my weekly medical column back in 2007 describing the experience of a reader, Mr Roger Andrews, in his mid-seventies. Five years earlier he had undergone a successful operation to repair an aortic aneurysm – which, astutely, he had self-diagnosed after noting a pronounced rhythmical pulsation in his abdomen while lying in bed one night. Subsequently, however, things had not gone well. He had become increasingly decrepit, immiserated by pain and stiffness in his legs that his doctors were unable to explain and which did not improve with anti-inflammatory pills. He was, however, determined to attend his son's wedding in Hawaii – not an easy journey, requiring him to use a wheelchair at the transfer stopovers. When reaching his destination, he realised he had forgotten to pack his cholesterol-lowering statins but was so vastly improved after the three weeks of not taking them he was able, on his return, to walk unassisted back through the terminal at Heathrow Airport. This brief account of the near miraculous restoration of his health and wellbeing prompted a deluge of correspondence from others with similar experiences of terrible side effects who were rewarded, after discontinuing their medication, by a similarly felicitous outcome.

'My husband gradually lost his energy during the eighteen months he was taking statins. He would come in from the garden and slump in a chair (quite unheard of) and I could outwalk him on walking holidays, particularly on hills (also quite unheard of). We put it down to anno domini – and at least we could walk comfortably together without me having to beg for a rest! Last September he got a very nasty tummy bug which lasted two weeks and during this time he stopped all his pills. Lo and behold, when he recovered, his energy level had returned and he has been back to normal ever since – minus his statins. His GP conceded his protracted debility could have been a side effect but had not warned him of the danger.'

Next, a woman in her mid-sixties, taking three different drugs (aspirin, beta blockers and a statin) since a heart attack eight years earlier, who similarly attributed her chronic ill health to 'increasing age':

'For a few years now, I have suffered from insomnia, ongoing tiredness every day, thinning hair, weakness in my leg muscles and, just recently, unhealing itchy rashes in sweaty parts of my body. Most worrying of all was the memory loss and the diminution of my hitherto substantial skills in creative writing. I thought most of these troubles were attributable to increasing age, but reading your column made me begin to think those troubles might be due to the statin I was taking. A month ago, I went to my doctor who agreed to let me take a statin holiday. I now sleep well, my only experience of tiredness is that which might be expected from my regained active lifestyle. My rashes are clearing up and my hair is regaining a little more lift in volume. My memory has improved greatly (I can once again bring the requisite word or fact to mind quickly), and my creative writing skills are returning. I hope for further strengthening in my leg muscles and my health in general to improve yet more.'

These – when one thinks about it – truly astonishing stories are recounted with an almost surprising lack of the recrimination one might expect from those who have taken a drug in the good faith that it would be beneficial, only to find it had precisely the contrary effect. Rather, the tone is almost matter-of-fact and completely persuasive. Now, like all family doctors, I vividly recall the therapeutic mishaps inadvertently inflicted on my patients – the skin rashes or diarrhoea from a course of antibiotics that may not have been strictly necessary, internal bleeding from anti-inflammatory drugs and similar misfortunes. But here, it seemed, such mishaps were much more prevalent than we family doctors realised.

Since the initial response to Mr Andrews's miracle cure, I have become only too aware through the experiences of thousands of readers of my medical column of the scale and ramifications of that 'hidden' epidemic of iatrogenic illness. And with it has come a recognition of a darker side – this is not just a matter of doctors prescribing 'too many pills', but one of coercing their patients into taking medicines they may not need and being defensively obtuse about the side effects that sometimes result.

The misfortunes of a woman in her mid-sixties deprived for eight years of the joys of climbing her beloved Lakeland fells through the over-zealous treatment of her mildly raised blood pressure illuminates this theme of 'doctors behaving badly':

'When my GP found I had mild raised blood pressure he started me on diuretic tablets once a day. On complaining of light-headedness and a general feeling of malaise, I was told I must take them or else I might have a stroke. Then I started getting muscle cramps in my legs and spent a fortune on private sports clinics. After eighteen months, the pain spread to my back and my physiotherapist suggested the diuretic might be depleting my body of salts and advised I discuss this further with my family doctor. His only response was to say that I had had sixty-eight active years and should find something less active to do. As an enthusiastic walker, skier, gardener and Scottish country dancer, I didn't find this satisfactory. I could hardly climb stairs, never mind a mountain. I eventually decided to stop the pills and bought a home blood pressure monitor and discovered the readings were volatile depending on how busy I was, but rarely above 155/70. I might add that, within a fortnight, my activities returned to normal and I can once again climb the fells.'

There is more indication of 'doctors behaving badly' in their refusal to discuss, and indeed their tendency to deny, the possibility that these drugs might have adverse effects. This from a previously energetic 58-year-old woman whose hobbies included long-distance horse riding and 'walking my dogs for miles each day':

'I was eventually frightened into taking statins by my GP three years ago when I could not get my cholesterol level below 7. When I asked him what the side effects might be he answered, "You will live longer." The actual side effects were . . . lack of energy . . . insomnia . . . weight gain . . . aching joints, all of which I put down to "the ageing process" and my whole life went into slow motion. I eventually chucked them away and two weeks later have regained my energy, sleep like the proverbial log, have lost 5lbs (due to the regained energy) and any muscle aches are now caused by my tearing around like a teenager jumping on and off horses, etc.'

Or again, 'Most of the doctors agree I am taking too many pills,' writes a man on thirteen different medications (including atorvastatin, Adizem, metformin, Monomil, omeprazole, doxazosin, finasteride, fluticasone, glimepiride and frusemide), 'but no one suggests stopping any of them.' He then describes the classic symptoms of polypharmacy-induced iatrogenic illness:

'I experience pain in my joints and muscle weakness as well as extreme lethargy. I also feel cold even when the sun is shining or the heating is on in the house. I am tired just walking a short distance and rarely leave the house except for medical appointments. I tend to fall asleep when I sit down to watch the TV. My hands recently started to shake and I find it difficult to lift anything heavier than half a bag of shopping.

This deterioration seems to have come on over the past year, prior to this I was able to get about and do jobs such as mow the lawn. I also used to go swimming, play tennis and attend a weekly exercise class.'

When the doctor does concede that one or other of the drugs being taken is the culprit, the insouciance with which he or she advises it be discontinued naturally raises the question of why it was prescribed in the first place – as with a woman in her early eighties following two severe falls, the result of a precipitous drop in her blood pressure caused by her medication:

'I have had two nasty falls. I just went down and hit my fore-head. Nothing broken. Two black eyes and a huge lump. I felt so unwell my doctor took me off all tablets, saying there was little difference in my blood pressure whether I was on them or not. I feel much better now.'

And again, a longish account from Edinburgh that encapsulates many of the issues already mentioned:

'My pre-op check for a varicose vein operation on my left leg revealed my blood pressure was very high (180/120). I was put on amlodipine and lisinopril by my GP and statins were added as "Your cholesterol is high". I am a regular hill walker and cyclist and over the next few months became very concerned as my stamina was disappearing. I gave up my weekly ride with the cycle club as I could no longer keep up, although I continued to go walking. I explained this to my GP and asked her, "Is there any possibility that the drugs I am on are responsible for this?" She said "No." Some months later my prescription was assessed by a pharmacist at the health centre. I asked her the same question and got the same answer.

I then began to get severe cramps in my neck during the night (every night), round about 1 a.m. Each morning I felt that I had been half strangled and had very limited neck movement. It was at this point I did some Googling and found reference to other side effects including muscle cramps. Ah ha! A light went on in my brain. 11 p.m., take simvastatin. 1 a.m., get cramps. This seemed more than a coincidence. That night I did not take the drug, bingo, no cramps. I had a GP check-up arranged for three weeks later and, having had no more cramps, told her that I would not be taking the statins again. She said, "Never mind, your cholesterol was not very high anyway." I was speechless. Over the next six months my stamina came back and I was eventually able to resume my cycling although have not fully recovered to the same level.'

These striking accounts, with many further variations (as will be seen), are powerful testimony to the 'hidden' problems of polypharmacy-induced iatrogenic illness. Their incidence is bound to be much greater than most family doctors appreciate, as GPs are disinclined, in their busy surgeries, to inquire too closely about the side effects of the drugs they prescribe – unless prompted to do so. Back in 1979, almost forty years ago, Derbyshire family doctor Cedrick Martys resolved to investigate the prevalence of iatrogenic illness in his practice. Over a period of two years he asked all his patients to whom he had prescribed a drug for the first time to fill in a simple questionnaire 'stating in their own words whether any symptoms occurring since starting treatment might have been a side effect of the drug received'. This is scarcely rocket science, but Dr Martys' findings were astonishing, with 40 per cent of his patients reporting symptoms – nausea, dizziness, fatigue, etc. – that could 'certainly' or 'probably' be attributed to the drug he had prescribed.

The rise of polypharmacy since Dr Martys conducted his study would suggest that this surprisingly high prevalence of drug-induced symptoms must by now be vastly greater. But it is only possible to *infer* this must be the case because, astonishingly – scandalously, one might think – no one knows. Put another way, that dizzying upward spiral in prescribing has occurred in almost complete ignorance of the true scale of the harms that might result. It does seem an extraordinary aberration, given all that is known about the side effects of medication, spelt out in almost excruciating detail in that hefty *Textbook of Iatrogenic Disease*, that doctors should have endorsed a programme of mass medication without any formal means of monitoring its potentially adverse consequences.

Still there is considerable circumstantial evidence of the scale of those 'adverse consequences' in the 75 per cent rise in emergency hospital admissions for 'adverse drug reaction' mentioned in the Introduction. The probability that polypharmacy is also implicated in the recently noted fall-off in life expectancy requires some elaboration. Throughout the twentieth century, and excepting the havoc caused by two world wars, life expectancy increased almost year by year, attributed variously to social factors (such as better housing and nutrition) and to medical progress, notably antibiotics that effectively abolished high infant mortality from infectious illness. Between 2000 and 2012 life expectancy increased by a further three years in Britain (and similarly in France, Germany and Italy) but then plateaued. And then the trend reversed, with a rising mortality rate in the older age groups – particularly in those aged eighty-five and beyond. Put simply, more people are dying than would be expected: an additional 600 a week, 30,000 a year in 2015 compared to the previous year.

The same phenomenon has been observed in other Western European countries and the United States, prompting much speculation as to what the explanation might be. It could just be a 'blip' in that upward trend in longevity, which could scarcely be expected to continue indefinitely. Several commentators have attributed it to 'austerity', the cuts in social spending that followed the financial crisis of 2008 – and indeed there is a precedent in the striking fall in life expectancy in the years immediately following the collapse of the Soviet Union, caused by increased alcoholism and suicide rates. This, however, could scarcely account for the consistency of the trends in Britain and elsewhere for which the rise in polypharmacy over the previous decade is a more plausible explanation, causing untimely death in several ways – as suggested by physician Dr Ian Scott's account of several instances of a Lazarus-type recovery from what would otherwise have been a fatal medication-induced illness. They include a woman in her nineties admitted to hospital almost moribund with low blood pressure (80/60) and acute kidney failure from the three different types of blood pressure-lowering medication she was taking. Her medication discontinued, she made a full recovery and returned home on 'no treatment' (she had previously been taking seven different drugs).

There is, as might be supposed, no simple explanation for this aberration of mass medicalisation which, as will be seen, stretches back four decades, orchestrated and effected by the synergistic (if at times unwitting) role of the three main 'players': the pharmaceutical industry, epidemiologists and general practitioners. I shall turn now briefly to examine each.

The pharmaceutical industry

Drug companies have become immensely rich and powerful by being smart, far-sighted and engaging at times in dodgy practices. We are (or certainly should be) aware of their contribution to transforming our lives immeasurably for the better with the discovery, in a few short decades after the war, of thousands of novel chemical compounds effective against the whole range of human tribulation – infectious diseases (obviously), circulatory disorders (heart attacks and stroke), mental afflictions (anxiety, depression, bipolar disorder), the painful swollen joints of rheumatic conditions, skin complaints such as psoriasis, inflammatory disorders of the gut (Crohn's disease and ulcerative colitis), cancer, and all the rest. But by the late seventies, when the cornucopia of novel drugs flowing from their research laboratories began to falter, they resorted to more devious means to maintain their profitability – catalogued in a shelf full of highly critical books with such self-explanatory titles as *Selling Sickness: How the World's Biggest Pharmaceutical*

Companies are Turning Us All into Patients; *Overtreated: How Too Much Medicine is Making Us Sicker and Poorer*; *Overdosed America*; *Our Daily Meds: How the Pharmaceutical Companies Transformed Themselves into Slick Marketing Machines and Hooked the Nation on Prescription Drugs*, and most influential of all, *The Truth About the Drug Companies, How they Deceive Us and What to Do About It* by Dr Marcia Angell, chief editor of the most prestigious of all US medical journals, the *New England Journal of Medicine*.

The insight that more than anything else would salvage the industry's fortunes was the realisation, as mentioned in the Introduction, that its future prosperity entailed moving beyond the development of drugs to combat disease by creating a market where they could 'sell to everyone' – targeting the hundreds of millions of the apparently well and healthy, persuading them (and indeed their doctors) that they had some medical condition warranting treatment. The most obvious way this might be achieved was to re-designate previously 'normal' physiological variables as 'abnormal', widening the net of those requiring lifelong medication with blood pressure and cholesterol-lowering drugs. They would, of course, have to demonstrate the efficacy of those drugs for this much wider market – a task likely to prove difficult, as the benefits for any individual were likely to be very small. So the necessary clinical trials had to be organised on a massive scale, involving thousands of patients and stretching over several years. Big trials cost big money and the only institutions with the necessary resources were the drug companies themselves, who thus became judge and jury of the merits of their own drugs. To recoup their substantial financial investment it was essential the results of those trials should be favourable – as indeed invariably they proved to be. And so it has come about, as Marcia Angell observes, that the pharmaceutical industry 'has moved very far from its original high purpose of discovering and producing useful new drugs. Now principally a marketing machine to sell drugs of dubious benefit, it uses its vast wealth and power to co-opt every institution that might stand in its way, including the Drug Regulatory Authorities, Academic Medical Centres – and the medical profession itself.'

The subterfuge and sleight of hand by which the industry has successfully portrayed its drugs to be vastly more effective than they really are will be considered later. It is, however, of interest to note here that over the past few years many of the major companies have been required to pay financial penalties varying from hundreds of millions to billions of dollars for corrupt and fraudulent practices (see Table 1.1). The scale of those fines would indicate their crimes were not trivial.

Table 1.1 The fines imposed on drug companies for corrupt and illegal practices 2007–2012

2008	Merck	$670 million
2009	Pfizer	$2.3 billion
	Eli Lilly	$1.4 billion
2010	Novartis	$423 million
	Astra Zeneca	$520 million
2011	GSK	$3 billion
2012	Johnson & Johnson	$1.1 billion
	Abbott	$1.5 billion

The epidemiologists

Who or what are epidemiologists? Most epidemiologists, though medically qualified, do not practise medicine; their skill lies rather in the deployment of statistical methods to identify the causes of disease and assess the benefits, or otherwise, of treatment. For many of us statistics are numbers to which complex mathematical formulae are applied to produce conclusions of dubious veracity from which all wit and common sense is rigorously excluded. Certainly, any single statistic by itself is a dreary thing, but when they are linked together over months and years, then patterns begin to emerge and it is possible to see things that previously were hidden. An unarguable event such as death lends itself particularly well to the statistical method, and when the numbers of deaths in any town or region are recorded over a period, it is possible to appreciate that in the aggregate they represent the distinct biological phenomenon of an epidemic. This – literally the study of epidemics – is the simplest form of epidemiology. Nonetheless, it has the power to change the world for the better.

Its origins stretch back to the movement for sanitary reform in the nineteenth century and the demonstration of the yawning differential in childhood mortality between the rich and poor. But its ascendancy to its current very influential role really begins in 1950 when the British epidemiologist Sir Austin Bradford Hill made in a single year two profound contributions to modern medicine. He deployed statistical methods first to prove unequivocally that smoking causes lung cancer and, second, to demonstrate that the most certain way of testing the efficacy of a drug is within the context of a clinical trial comparing the outcome in those given the treatment with that in others given a placebo.

It is impossible to exaggerate the significance of these two instances of 'revealing what was previously hidden': not only did they prove that this commonest and most deadly of cancers is preventable (by not smoking), they provided the 'gold standard' by which the efficacy of every form of medical intervention could be rigorously assessed.

Still, statistics can be tricky, and epidemiologists nowadays do not necessarily deploy them with Sir Austin's degree of intellectual probity. They have, as it were, played the role of handmaiden to the pharmaceutical industry in promoting their goal of 'selling to everyone' in three different ways. The first, as mentioned in the Introduction, is the proposition that the 'population is sick', the mean or average of those three variables blood pressure, cholesterol and glucose is too high and there is more to be gained by lowering it in everyone than by focusing on those at high risk.

Next, in the 1980s, epidemiologists convinced themselves, and sought to persuade all of us, that the foods we enjoy – notably meat, milk and dairy products – are the primary cause of most common illnesses (heart disease, stroke and cancer), which are preventable by switching to a 'healthier' diet with an emphasis on bread, pasta, potatoes and other high carbohydrate foods. Specifically, the powerful imagery of how 'high fat' foods increase the levels of cholesterol in the blood, and thus the risk of heart disease, would become the stalking horse for the drug companies' promotion of the near-universal prescription of their staggeringly profitable cholesterol-lowering statins. The third contribution of epidemiologists to the promotion of mass medication has been their favourable interpretation of the outcome of those drug company-sponsored clinical trials.

General practitioners

The last of the players, I am sad to say, are my fellow general practitioners, who in 2004 did a Faustian deal with the government, sacrificing their professional independence for the financial gain of being 'paid for performance'. Now, generously rewarded for their success in hitting targets of numbers of patients treated, they are – if unintentionally – deeply complicit in that 'hidden' epidemic of iatrogenic illness.

The synergistic contribution of these three 'players' to the rise of polypharmacy is deeply embedded within routine medical practice with not the slightest chance it will be reversed in the foreseeable future. Thus, the only way for people to escape the clutches of 'too much medicine' is, as suggested, by taking the initiative themselves through an understanding of the arguments and the evidence that sustains it. But that surely is impossible. The relevant evidence in favour of (and indeed against) the current policy of mass medication is vast, far beyond the comprehension of any individual, a library's worth at least of epidemiological studies and thousands of clinical trials involving tens of thousands of patients in which the relevant drugs have been investigated. Still, if intriguingly, the crux of the matter can be reduced to a few simple graphs and the elementary application of common sense to numbers. *Pour encourager*, here is a preview.

The first is a striking graph of the rise and fall of heart disease in the United States over a period of sixty years, increasing incrementally year by year, peaking, and then exhibiting a similarly precipitous fall (Figure 1.2). This is clearly not the pattern of an illness strongly determined by social factors, such as major changes in food preferences – for were it to be so, as the epidemiologists maintain, that would have required that sometime in the early twentieth century everyone almost simultaneously adopted an 'unhealthy' diet (to account for the rise), then in the early sixties switched back to a 'healthy' diet (to account for the fall). This did not happen. Cholesterol, as will be seen, may not be entirely innocent but the epidemiologists who assert its determinant role

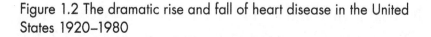

Figure 1.2 The dramatic rise and fall of heart disease in the United States 1920–1980

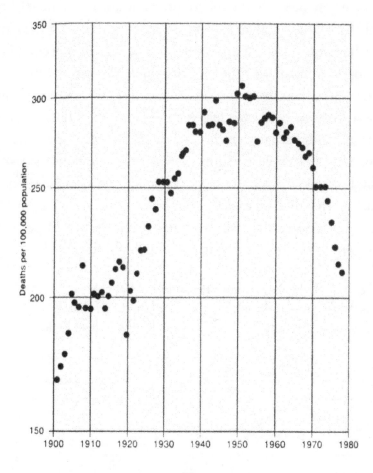

in causing heart disease must be in error – and thus, as will be seen, the rationale for the mass prescription of those cholesterol-lowering statin drugs is deeply undermined.

Next is the mischief by which drugs are persistently and mis-leadingly portrayed as being much more effective than they really are. Most would readily agree to take a drug that reduced by 20 per cent their chance of having a fatal heart attack – as claimed for the first of the cholesterol-lowering drugs, cholestyramine. It would seem foolish not to – and there it is in black and white: –20 per cent on the upper of the two rows in Table 1.2. But immediately below is the much more modest figure of –0.4 per cent that is the 'absolute' benefit for the person taking the drug. In other words, for every hundred people, it will prevent a fatal coronary in just 0.4 of them – or (which amounts to the same thing) more than two hundred people must take cholestyramine (not a pleasant drug) for five years to save one life from heart disease. And that puts a rather different gloss on matters: for the remaining 199, cholestyramine, rather than reducing the risk of a fatal coronary by 20 per cent, will make zero difference as to whether they live or die. Or, put another way, the claim that the drug reduces the risk of a fatal coronary by '20 per cent' exaggerates the true worth to the individual fifty-fold.

Table 1.2 The numbers game: The 'relative' benefits of cholestyramine in reducing the risk of a fatal heart attack is fifty times greater than the 'absolute' benefit for the individual taking it

	Cardiac deaths
Relative rate reduction	–20%
Absolute rate reduction	–0.4%

This deception is universal as neither drug companies nor doctors could hope to persuade anyone to take a drug for so trivial a benefit. The alchemy by which the molehill of 'absolute risk reduction' is transformed into the mountain of 'relative risk reduction' is, as will be seen, very easy to grasp and, once done, permits anyone to make a properly informed decision about the medical advice they receive. So that is all it takes – one (very striking) graph and a couple of figures – to realise that there is something deeply fishy about the rise of polypharmacy that demands clarification.

A final word

In the words of G. K. Chesterton, 'History is a high point of advantage from which alone we can see the age in which we live.' And it is only from the high point of advantage of understanding the historical origins of polypharmacy that we can properly appreciate the blight it inflicts on so many lives. This book, then, is written as an historical narrative, its several interconnecting themes emerging ever more clearly as it progresses. The penultimate chapter, 'Oldies – The Great Betrayal', and the two appendices, 'Fractured Follies' and 'The (Toxic) Cardiac Cocktail', will be of particular interest, respectively, to those in their seventies and beyond and to those taking preventive medication for osteoporosis and taking the cocktail of drugs routinely prescribed following procedures on the heart. We start with how it all began: 'The Triumph of Prevention'.

Chapter 2

The Triumph of Prevention

There is no more certain way of maximising the chances of living as long as possible (besides, of course, not smoking) than every so often dropping in to see the family doctor to have one's blood pressure checked and – if found to be elevated – taking regular medication to lower it. For, as everyone knows, raised blood pressure left untreated may burst a blood vessel in the brain. The catastrophic complications, if not lethal, include paralysis, loss of speech, and many other highly undesirable variations of functional impairment – the prospect of which was brought home to me with considerable urgency soon after my fiftieth birthday.

My first intimation something was seriously amiss came when, in the bath one evening, I was puzzled to note the water around my left leg seemed a lot cooler than around my right. It was not, of course. The temperature of the bath was uniform but my left leg had lost the ability to discriminate between hot and cold. This prompted a sleepless night wondering whether I might have unwittingly had a stroke affecting the relevant parts of the brain, or whether this might even be the premonitory sign of something even more sinister, such as a brain tumour. I was thus more than relieved that a CT brain scan revealed nothing seriously amiss and, as my friendly neurologist suggested, the loss of sensitivity to heat must be due to disturbed functioning of the sensory nerves, perhaps caused by a viral infection, in my lower spine – for which there was nothing to be done but which would, with luck, improve with time. I would, however, have to attend to my blood pressure of (alarmingly) 180/115 – with a 99 per cent certainty of my experiencing some serious or indeed fatal misfortune such as a stroke, heart attack, kidney or heart failure by the time I was sixty-five.

The unequivocal evidence that this gloomy prospect can be prevented ranks among the most significant of all the many achievements of modern medicine. This is the triumph of prevention. The absence of effective treatment for hypertension prior to the 1960s had a profound effect not just on individuals but on the fate of whole nations. Both the President of the United States, Franklin D. Roosevelt, and the Russian leader, Josef Stalin, had raised blood pressure, with profound consequences for world politics in the post-war years. On 12 April 1945 Roosevelt died of a cerebral haemorrhage which his physician, Admiral Ross McIntire, said had 'come out of the clear sky', as only a few days earlier the President had apparently been 'given a thorough examination by eight physicians including some of the most eminent in the country and pronounced physically sound in every way'. The admiral was lying. Roosevelt had been diagnosed as having severe hypertension almost ten years earlier, which by the time of the Yalta conference with Churchill and Stalin in February 1945 (just eight weeks before his death) had caused so much damage to his heart and kidneys that he was 'a dying man'. At this crucial moment in world politics, Roosevelt's ailing health so impaired his political judgement as to produce 'a deadly hiatus' in the leadership of the United States that would lead to 'the betrayal of the Poles, the imposition of communist governments in Eastern Europe, the Czechoslovakian coup and – on the other side of the world – the loss of China and the invasion of South Korea'.

Eight years later, in 1953, Stalin also fell victim to a stroke, at the age of seventy-three. Again, the history of the post-war world would have been very different if his hypertension had been treatable with appropriate medication. He could well have lived on for another decade, up to and including the Cuban missile crisis, which might then have had a very different outcome, culminating in the Soviet Union, under his psychotic leadership, launching a full-scale nuclear war against the United States. One way or another, hypertension has had a crucial impact on the fate of nations. So how did it become treatable?

The term 'blood pressure' refers to the pressure generated by the contraction of the heart muscle to pump blood into the arteries and around the circulatory system. A normal reading for an otherwise healthy middle-aged person is around 130 (systolic)/80 (diastolic), the latter being the more significant – the higher the diastolic pressure, the greater the risk of stroke. This blood pressure is influenced by two factors. The first is the volume of blood in the arteries (the higher the volume, the greater the pressure needed to pump it round the circulation), and the second the diameter of the vessels through which the blood travels (the narrower the arteries, the greater the pump-ing pressure that is required). Hence, prior to the discovery of effective drugs, the only two ways of lowering the blood pressure were either to reduce the volume of fluid in the circulatory system or to dilate the blood vessels.

In 1944 a German-born physician at Duke University, Dr Walter Kempner, reported that blood pressure could be returned to 'normal or almost normal' by reducing the volume of fluid in the circulatory system with a rice/fruit/sugar diet: 'The rice boiled or steamed in plain water without salt, milk or fat. Fruit juices and fruit are allowed with the exception of nuts, dates, avocados, and any kind of dried or tinned fruit. No water is allowed and the fluid intake is restricted to one litre of fruit juice per day.' The problem, as can be imagined, was that the diet itself was so unpalatable that patients could not stick with it. 'It is insipid, unappetising and monotonous and demands great care in its preparation ... it is quite impracticable for a member of a large household with minimal domestic help as its deadly monotony tends to make it intolerable unless the physician can infuse into the patient some of the asceticism of the religious zealot.'

The second approach to treating hypertension – dilating the diameter of the arteries so less pressure is required to push the blood around the body – involved an operation to cut the nerves that control the diameter of the arteries in the legs (a bilateral lumbar sympathectomy). This operation was a major procedure and thus limited to those who were still fairly fit and young.

The limitations of these treatments are self-evident and with severe hypertension being a lifelong illness, its complications only became truly preventable with the development, just over sixty years ago, of drugs sufficiently well tolerated they can be taken indefinitely. In the post-war years, research chemists in the burgeoning pharmaceutical industry sought a chemical compound that might fulfil this role. And here they could scarcely have been more successful, producing, at the latest count, more than ten different classes of drugs each capable of lowering the blood pressure in a different way – diuretics, beta blockers, calcium channel blockers, ACE inhibitors, etc., with numerous variations of each – a total of eighty different drugs in all. The almost unbelievable benefit they confer was dramatically demonstrated in a study of just 140 US veterans with a diastolic pressure (like my own) of 115 or above allocated to take either a blood pressure-lowering drug or placebo. Within just eighteen months the study was discontinued, as the merits of lowering the blood pressure were so striking (see Table 2.1) that it would have been unethical to continue to deny

Table 2.1 The triumph of prevention: The unequivocal benefit of treatment in preventing the complications of severe hypertension in the Veterans' Administration trial

Outcome	No Treatment (Control)	Treatment (Intervention)
Death	4	0
Stroke	4	1
Heart failure	4	0
Heart attack	2	0
Kidney failure	3	0
Eye haemorrhage	7	0
Hospitalised for high blood pressure	3	0
Treatment complication	0	1
Total	27	2

the drug to those in the placebo group. It is scarcely necessary to emphasise the significance of just how badly the latter had fared: compared to all the zeros in the treatment column, 38 per cent (twenty-seven out of the seventy) sustained one or other of the well-known complications of severe hypertension – stroke, heart failure, heart attack and so on. And it is further possible to predict that, without treatment, that figure of 38 per cent would over the next five years have risen to 80 per cent and after ten years to 99 per cent. Put another way, for those with severe hypertension, most, if not quite all these catastrophes can be avoided by taking blood pressure-lowering medication – making it probably the single most successful of all medical interventions.

This unequivocal verdict transformed, as can be imagined, the everyday practice of medicine, providing the strongest possible incentive for doctors to widen the scope of their concerns to systematically seek out among the legions of their seemingly healthy patients those with markedly raised blood pressure – and to be rewarded in their endeavours by the satisfaction of the certainty of doing so much good. For myself, fifteen years on, popping my pills out of their silver foil every morning has long since become a holy ritual, so secure a guarantee of my present and future health that I feel distinctly uneasy if, for any reason, I omit to take them.

So far, so straightforward. But widening the domain of medicine by identifying and treating those with severe hypertension certainly does not prevent all those strokes, heart attacks and so on, many of which occur in those whose blood pressure is only modestly elevated. The reason for this perhaps surprising paradox requires clarification. Taking one million people at random, measuring their blood pressure will produce a bell-shaped curve where most with a diastolic pressure of 80 or less are in the middle (at the top of the bell, as it were) fading away on either side to the low or the very high (115 or more) (as shown in Figure 2.1).

Figure 2.1 The bell-shaped curve of the proportion of the adult population with a high, normal and low blood pressure

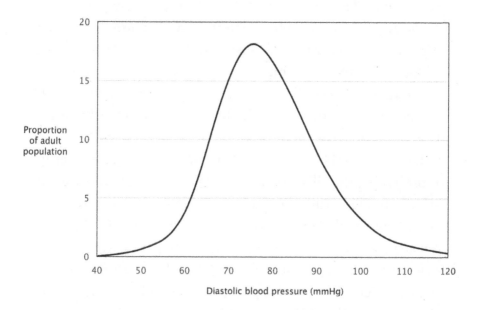

Now, predictably the risk of stroke gradually rises starting from the base line of the mean (or 'average') diastolic pressure of 80, increasing two-fold at 95 to more than five-fold at 110 or above. The crux of the matter is the degree to which the unequivocal evidence of benefit of treating the few (1.2 per cent) with severe hypertension (a diastolic pressure of more than 115) extends to the many (25 per cent) in whom it is modestly elevated ('mild' hypertension) – bearing in mind that this would vastly expand the numbers on medication. Self-evidently, the risk of stroke being so much lower in those with mild hypertension, the chances for the individual of benefiting from treatment will be considerably less – but by how much?

The size of the clinical trial necessary to answer this crucial question gives some sense of what is at stake here. It took just 140 patients to demonstrate the prodigious benefits of treating severe hypertension, but more than 17,000 patients to answer the same question in those with mild hypertension in a trial organised by the Medical Research Council (MRC) in the 1980s, comparing the outcome in patients with a diastolic pressure of between 90 and 110 given no treatment with those treated with either a thiazide diuretic (bendrofluazide) or a beta blocker (propranolol).

Come the end of the study, there were fifty fewer strokes in those 'taking the pills' (Table 2.2). This would seem very useful; still, it is interesting to note, by contrast with that veterans trial, how small a proportion of the participants in this trial apparently benefited from medication – 2.6 per cent of those on placebo had a stroke compared to 1.4 per cent of those on the pills, a difference of just 1.2 per cent. Put another way, medication improves the chances of not having a stroke in those with mild hypertension from 97.4 per cent to 98.6 per cent.

Furthermore, perhaps surprisingly, lowering the blood pressure does not seem to confer any overall advantage. As will also be noted, there is almost no difference in the numbers dying, whether on treatment (248) or taking the placebo (253). From this it is possible to calculate that it is necessary to treat 850 patients with mild hypertension for a year to prevent the chances

Table 2.2 The 'important but infrequent benefit' of treating mild hypertension in the MRC trial

	Placebo	Rate %	BP Lowering medication	Rate %
Strokes	109	2.6	60	1.4
Heart attack	234	5.4	222	5.2
Deaths from all causes	253	5.9	248	5.8

of one of them having a stroke – 'an important but infrequent benefit'. Meanwhile – and again in marked contrast to those veterans with severe hypertension – the chances of being alive after five years are the same as for those not taking any medication.

Even the modest benefit of preventing one stroke for every 850 people treated is more modest still when applied to the 'real world' of everyday medical practice. Blood pressure, as all know, fluctuates throughout the day and rises in response to visiting the doctor (so-called 'white coat' hypertension), or to the stress of trouble at work, bereavement and so on. Hence the necessity, prior to diagnosing someone as having raised blood pressure, to measure it on several occasions. This rigmarole may be mandatory in the context of a clinical trial but is less frequently adhered to in everyday practice, with the inevitable result that hypertension is 'over-diagnosed' – which in turn explains why for one in ten of those so diagnosed, their blood pressure remains within the normal range when their medication is discontinued. And those over-diagnosed as having hypertension will, by definition, not benefit from being treated. Thus, 'in the real world', family doctors may be treating as many as a thousand people for every stroke prevented.

Still, the debacle of a stroke is best avoided. So why not take the pills in the hope of being the one in a thousand who might benefit from doing so? But the doctors who had devoted so much time and energy to mounting the MRC trial (in the confident expectation its results would be more favourable) were not even certain about that, noting the 'important but infrequent' benefit of medication subjected a substantial proportion 'to chronic side effects most, but not all, minor'. Those adverse effects, sufficiently serious for some to warrant stopping their drugs, were – for those on bendrofluazide – impotence (20 per cent of men), gout (12 per cent), diabetes (10 per cent); and – for propranolol – lethargy (10 per cent), shortness of breath (8 per cent), nausea and dizziness (7 per cent) and Raynaud's phenomenon of cold hands and feet (6 per cent).

This subtle pay-off between benefits and risks, one might imagine, should have encouraged a cautious attitude as to the level of blood pressure that warranted the use of drugs to lower it. But, on the contrary, in the thirty years since that definitive MRC trial, millions more have been so labelled, the number rising remorselessly from one in ten to one in four adults (and more than 70 per cent of 'oldies'), paralleled by a sky-rocketing eight-fold increase in prescription for antihypertensives, from 8 million in 1985 to 63 million in 2007. How did that come about?

This brings us to the most astonishing – in its implications, at least – medical theory of the twentieth century: the 'population approach', touched on in the Introduction and Chapter 1 – the proposition that there is more to be gained from treating the blood pressure in the millions with mild hypertension than in the relatively few (like myself) in whom it is markedly raised. This theory, first proposed by prominent epidemiologist

Professor Geoffrey Rose in his article 'Sick individuals and sick populations', runs as follows. Self-evidently, it is as (more or less) sick individuals that we seek medical attention, consulting the family doctor in the hope that he or she will identify the cause of, for example, a severe episode of back pain or a puzzling skin rash and prescribe the appropriate medication to correct it. The same principle can be extended to those like myself, who though subjectively healthy have severe hypertension, in the near certainty that treatment will do good by preventing some otherwise inevitable catastrophe.

But, as already noted from observing the bell curve of the distribution of blood pressure, many strokes also occur in the millions whose blood pressure is normal or only mildly raised. Thus, Rose argued, one could say that everyone – the whole population – was 'sick', that a diastolic pressure of 90 was in fact too high and that lowering it by some simple means, in effect shifting that bell curve leftward (Figure 2.2), would thus significantly reduce the number of strokes.

This concept is admittedly difficult to grasp, but may be more readily understood in relation to another issue Professor Rose considered suitable for what he called his 'population strategy' – preventing the harmful effects of heavy drinking. There is, as with blood pressure, a bell-shaped curve of alcohol consumption, most people drinking modestly (the top of the bell curve) while the numbers fall off in one direction to a relatively small number of teetotallers and, in the other direction, to the extreme of heavy drinkers prone to all the physical and psychological problems associated with alcoholism – liver cirrhosis, nerve and brain damage, domestic violence and so on. Now the obvious – one might think the only – way of preventing such alcohol-induced damage is to provide the sort of rehabilitation

Figure 2.2 Shifting the bell-shaped curve to the left reduces the risk of stroke in 'the many' with a normal or slightly raised blood pressure

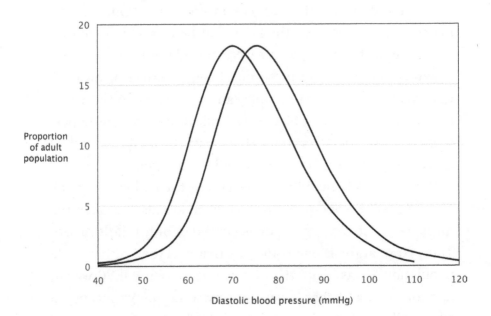

programmes that support heavy drinkers in their efforts to abstain from their injurious addiction. But Rose proposed (and here one has to concentrate a little because it is such an extraordinary concept) the problems associated with alcoholism would be more readily prevented were those millions of *moderate* drinkers to slightly reduce their alcohol consumption – by, say, one glass of wine a day. This would theoretically reduce the 'average' consumption, and by shifting the overall distribution leftwards would result in reducing the number of heavy drinkers at the right end of the curve prone to all those physical and mental harms outlined above. The same logic applied to tackling obesity would be to focus attention on encouraging the modestly plump, rather than the seriously overweight, to go on a diet; thus the 'average' weight would fall and there would be fewer of the seriously obese at the top end of the distribution curve. And the same principle applied to preventing strokes is predicated on the supposition – a highly contentious one, as will be seen – that the amount of salt consumed is a major factor in raised blood pressure. Thus, Rose argued, were everyone to make small changes (such as not adding salt to their potatoes), this would then lower the average levels of blood pressure and thus markedly reduce the numbers of those, like myself, at 'high risk' of stroke because of their markedly raised blood pressure.

In summary, this 'population approach' to treatment (i.e. directed at the entire population), he argued, was likely to be more effective than just focusing on those with serious problems of alcoholism or obesity or markedly raised blood pressure, not just by 'shifting the distribution', and thus reducing the numbers that fall into these categories, but also by encompassing the millions at low risk – those with normal levels of alcohol consumption, blood pressure, etc. – as 'a large number of people at [minuscule] risk gives rise to more cases than the small number at high risk'. He conceded this would only confer a small benefit to each individual 'since most are going to be alright anyway', a phenomenon he dubbed the Prevention Paradox – 'A preventive measure which brings much benefit to the population offers little to each participating individual'.

Rose conceded he could not be certain this strategy would be effective in the way he anticipated. But, he wrote, 'Certainty is not a prerequisite for action ... A sick patient can expect from a physician only a reasonable confidence that the diagnosis is right and the treatment likely to do more good than harm. Prevention [by treating the population as "sick"] should be judged in the same way.'

Intuitively, however, any sensible person would know, without the advantages of being a professor of epidemiology, that this 'population strategy' must be fallacious. How could my drinking one glass of wine less a day conceivably influence the burden of alcoholism in society? Or how could others, by not adding salt to their potatoes, reduce the chances for someone like myself with severe hypertension of suffering a stroke?

And fallacious Professor Rose's strategy certainly is. Contradicted by the most elementary of considerations, it is predicated on the assumption that the 'normal' behaviour or physiological measurement of the *many* determines the prevalence of medical and social problems. Or, as Professor Rose himself expressed it, 'The population "mean" [i.e. the average alcohol consumption / blood pressure] *predicts* the number of "deviant" individuals' – where 'deviants' are those that differ from the norm by being overweight or alcoholic or having severe hypertension and so on. So, 'to help this minority of deviants, the majority must change'.

But it is scarcely necessary to point out 'the population' is not some single homogenous entity. The laws of natural biological variation ensure that everyone is different, a fact readily apparent from a stroll down the high street. Furthermore, the factors that might predispose to the 'deviancy' of alcoholism in one individual, such as a troubled childhood, are quite different from those of others where it might be due to an unhappy marriage, or genetic predisposition or depressive personality. Again, very small babies are 'deviant' in the sense that they weigh less than the norm, but the reasons are quite different depending on whether the smallness is due to their having been born prematurely, or to some environmental factor (such as their mother continuing to smoke during pregnancy), or indeed to genetics, where both parents are small.

The supposition that the 'average' blood pressure, weight or alcohol intake of the population can tell us something about the deviancy of hypertension, obesity or alcoholism, noted one of Professor Rose's critics, 'is analogous to claiming that the causes of gigantism or dwarfism can be discovered by studying people of normal height'.

Professor Rose's disregard for these elementary laws of biological variation that distinguish one person from another in favour of the statistical abstraction of the bell-shaped curve extends to his 'solution' – that of lowering the 'average' blood pressure by the simple expedient of everyone not adding salt to their potatoes. This is an impossibility, being contradicted – as every fifteen-year-old knows from his GCSE science lessons – by the phenomenon of homeostasis, where a multiplicity of different mechanisms combine to ensure that blood pressure remains stable within the same narrow limits, ensuring the constancy of the blood flow to the brain whether we are lying flat, standing or even standing on our heads. We could not survive otherwise. The corollary, as in Walter Kempner's 'insipid, unappetising and monotonous' diet mentioned above, is that it requires truly heroic (and unacceptable) dietary changes to lower the blood pressure.

For all that, Professor Rose's contention that the 'population is sick' and 'the majority must change to help the minority of deviants' proved to be (and remains) incredibly influential. Twenty years later another prominent epidemiologist, Professor Michael Marmot, claimed it to be 'now so widely accepted it is hard to realise how radical it was when first outlined . . . it has changed our whole approach to improving health.' How come? To be sure, Professor Rose's strategy is condemned by its biological implausibility and impracticality – with one important qualification: small dietary changes may not lower the blood pressure but drugs certainly do. The endorsement of the 'population approach' provided the theoretical rationale for the pharmaceutical industry to pursue its goal of mass medicalisation.

Over the next twenty years it would encourage hypertension experts to redefine the cut-off point for 'mild' hypertension down from 160/100 to include all those additional millions that were around the top of the bell curve with a blood pressure of 140/90 or above. How many of these really had 'hypertension' is uncertain for, as already noted, blood pressure varies markedly over time depending on the circumstances – as retired geriatrician Oscar Jolobe recalls, having visited his doctor soon after receiving a 'worrying' call from his solicitor.

'My blood pressure was recorded as 154/78. The following week I made a record of my home blood pressures and the thirty-one readings averaged 137/79. Subsequently I recorded it four to five times a day. All the standing systolic pressures fell within the range of 100–130 except for two occasions of 96 and 90 respectively.'

There is no knowing, then, how many doctors go through the rigmarole of measuring the blood pressure on several separate occasions to ensure it is indeed raised, especially when the financial incentives to GPs discourage them from doing so – as Lincolnshire GP Edmund Willis describes.

'We have two options in dealing with the massive number of patients with a mildly raised blood pressure reading.
    Option 1. We can diligently check the blood pressure many times, discuss lifestyle changes in detail [that, for example, it might fall were they to lose a few pounds in weight], and

arrange regular follow-ups at which we will have to go through the whole discussion again about treating or not treating with drugs.

Option 2. We can start the patient on drugs and treat the blood pressure according to protocol. If the patients get side effects that is the drugs' fault, not ours. We will also be paid more.'

And then, an initially raised blood pressure will subsequently fall back within the normal range, either without medication, as occurred in one-fifth of those allocated to receive the placebo in the MRC trial, or after their drugs are discontinued.

'It is all too often that a hospital doctor sees patients on one to three antihypertensives for the "good control" of their blood pressure,' observes Dr Jecko Thachil, Clinical Lecturer at the University of Liverpool. 'Their drugs are appropriately stopped and very often on discharge these medications are not recommenced on their take-home prescriptions.'

Now, the prompt initiation of drugs without first taking into account this variability of the blood pressure is not simply 'bad medicine' but also unethical. Treating someone with mild hypertension (however defined) is, after all, qualitatively different from treating a cough and fever due to a chest infection, where the doctor can reasonably assume implicit consent when prescribing a course of antibiotics in the certainty that it will be of immediate and direct advantage. By contrast, the same doctor initiating lifelong blood pressure-lowering medication should make clear the modest benefit of doing so. Here the principle of autonomy, the central principle of medical ethics, holds that individuals are entitled to make important decisions about their lives ('no decision about me, without me'). And, without doubt, that includes taking drugs indefinitely. Thus, the doctor, in recognising a patient's autonomy, should first obtain the patient's *informed* consent as to the benefits and risks of the antihypertensive drugs he prescribes. But they rarely do so. Rather, as will be recalled from the previous chapter, the Lakeland fell walker felt coerced into taking medication with the threat of being struck down by a stroke if she failed to do so. Meanwhile her suspicion that perhaps her drugs might be responsible for her debilitating symptoms ('I could scarcely climb the stairs let alone a mountain') was summarily dismissed.

Indeed, when informed consent is sought by explaining in a comprehensible way the findings of the MRC trial – 'Drugs have a 3 per cent chance of preventing a stroke but a 97 per cent chance of doing no good or not being needed in your case' – nearly half will decline to take them. The further reason it is necessary for doctors to seek informed consent is that all drugs will have some side effects in some people, the more so when they have to be taken indefinitely. The side effects of the more commonly prescribed antihypertensives are summarised in Table 2.3; their potential, when taken by millions, for causing much misery and suffering is obviously considerable.

It is, of course, difficult to imagine the scale of the distress such iatrogenic illness might inflict, but it is at least readily 'curable' by the simple expedient of discontinuing the drug responsible. This is, however, not necessarily straightforward, as the symptoms may be insidious or misattributed to 'getting on' ('What can you expect at your age?'). Two cautionary tales of the 'insidious' will illustrate the point. The first, the depletion of body salts (sodium and potassium) with a thiazide diuretic – as described by a woman in her mid-seventies:

'About six years ago, when attending hospital as a day case for an endoscopy, I was told my blood pressure was that of a 21-year-old. That was pleasing to hear – only to be told by my GP a few months later that my blood pressure was very high and I was prescribed bendrofluazide. I took it for about four years till one night both my legs started to ache simultaneously and I found it difficult to stand for even short periods.

A friend recommended a doctor who, it was said, was brilliant at diagnosing conditions that other doctors overlooked. A blood test revealed that the bendrofluazide had depleted the potassium in my body and it was advised I stop taking them

Table 2.3 The adverse effects of the four most commonly prescribed types of blood pressure-lowering drug

Thiazide Diuretics	ACE Inhibitors
Gout	Dry Irritating cough
Diabetes	Angioedema
Erectile dysfunction	Acute kidney failure
Sudden death	
	Beta Blockers
Calcium Channel Blockers	Wheezing
Headaches	Sleep disturbances
Palpitations	Fatigue
Flushing	Exercise intolerance
Gum hypertrophy	Erectile dysfunction
Heart failure	Raynaud's phenomenon
Constipation	Heart failure
Alopecia	Sudden death
Allergic drug reactions	

which I did and, as if by magic, my symptoms disappeared. I do still regularly have my blood pressure checked which, interestingly, is within the normal range without medication.'

Next, a gentleman who describes his experience since being prescribed the beta blocker bisoprolol:

'I have suffered tiredness, fainting on aeroplanes and "not feeling very lively". Recently, a local GP sent me to see a kidney specialist because I was suffering from "extreme tiredness syndrome". She turned out to be a real star and took a holistic view suggesting I purchase a blood pressure monitor, record the results for a few weeks and then see my own GP about possibly revising my medication. I duly did this and found that sometimes my blood pressure was as low as 100 (systolic) and my heart rate in the fifties. My GP agreed to reduce the dose and after a few days I started to feel much better and now feel significantly more "lively" (at least for a 71-year-old).'

Both thiazide diuretics and beta blockers can, it should be noted, cause 'sudden death' when a low potassium or slowing of the heart rate induces a potentially lethal disturbance of heart rhythm. It is impossible to say how frequently this may occur, as by definition such deaths will be unexplained or attributed to some other cause. The potentially fatal consequences of a treatment-induced precipitous drop in blood pressure (postural hypotension) are, however, well documented.

So, in summary, we started back in 1967 with the unequivocal findings of a small study of just 140 US veterans with severe hypertension to which, without exaggeration, I owe my life. This was followed eighteen years later by the considerably more equivocal results from the MRC trial of 17,000 patients with mild hypertension. That could have been a major disappointment for the pharmaceutical industry but, buttressed by Professor Rose's very influential 'population theory', they encouraged the experts to drive down the cut-off point for defining hypertension, thus expanding by millions the number of those deemed eligible for treatment. To take just one example, from Canada, between 1996 and 2006 the number of prescriptions for thiazide diuretics increased by 127 per cent, for beta blockers by 87 per cent, for calcium channel blockers by 55 per cent, for ACE inhibitors by 108 per cent and for the angiotensin receptor blockers by a startling 4,054 per cent.

This experiment in mass medicalisation inflicted on the population without their informed consent, with no 'certainty' it would be effective, has now been running for the best part of thirty years, providing sufficient time for a reasoned judgement as to its success or failure.

Let us return briefly to the MRC trial with that equivocal outcome of 'an important but infrequent benefit' where the merits of treating 850 (or more) individuals to avoid one person experiencing a stroke must be offset against the substantial risk of iatrogenic harm. The consequence of the progressive lowering of the threshold for diagnosing mild hypertension dictated by the 'population strategy', to include the millions whose blood pressure is in the range of 140–159/90–99, is that they now account for almost two-thirds (60 per cent) of those labelled as having 'hypertension'. The definitive verdict came in 2012 with a review of the several clinical trials comparing the merits of antihypertensive drugs with no treatment: 'Compared to placebo, treatment with antihypertensive drugs does not reduce any outcome', noted Professor Stephen Martin of the University of Massachusetts in an editorial in the *British Medical Journal*. 'It reduces neither stroke nor heart disease nor total mortality.' From this he concludes, 'It would be less costly [to the tune of $19 billion, the cost of treating mild hypertension in the United States] and yield better outcomes to target efforts in high risk patients rather than low risk individuals with unclear benefits.'

So much, then, for this particular application (there will be more) of Professor Rose's 'population strategy'. The financial cost is at least readily calculable, the burden of the iatrogenic illness it has caused, as noted, less so.

In Chapter 7, I shall examine the yet more grievous consequences of the over-treatment of hypertension in those in their seventies and beyond. But we turn now to the central pillar of polypharmacy – the mass prescription of cholesterol-lowering statins – the source of Roger Andrews's chronic decrepitude, as described in the previous chapter, that first alerted me to the scale of the hidden epidemic of iatrogenic illness.

The saga behind their near-universal prescription is truly extraordinary, stretching back over the past sixty years and predicated on two seemingly persuasive but erroneous epidemiological theories. The first, already encountered, is the 'population approach', the supposition that the 'normal' or average cholesterol level is too high and the necessity (as with the bell curve of blood pressure) to shift its distribution downwards by pharmacological means. This, of course, requires the incrimination of cholesterol as a primary determinant cause of heart disease. And here we encounter the second of those theories, the contentious, all-encompassing proposition that most common illnesses, such as heart attacks, can be attributed to the consumption of 'high fat' meat, milk and dairy products and are thus preventable by switching to a 'healthy' diet. This can seem a bit puzzling as heart disease has, after all, been around a long time. In the sixteenth century, Leonardo da Vinci, in his 'Anatomy of an Old Man', described the typical narrowing of the arteries with age when he spoke of 'debility from deficiency of the arteries that nourish the heart and the lower limbs'. Then in 1772, the English physician William Heberden succinctly described the characteristic crushing anginal pains of heart disease brought on by exertion:

'They who are afflicted with it are seized while they are walking, (more especially if it be uphill, and soon after eating) with a painful and most disagreeable sensation in the breast which seems as if it would extinguish life, if it were to increase or continue; but the moment they stand still, all this uneasiness vanishes.'

More than a century later, Russian physician Vladimir Kernig described two cases, confirmed at autopsy, of 'sudden death' due to the presence of a clot (or thrombus) in the arteries to the heart:

'The severe and prolonged paroxysms of angina pectoris may be explained by the presence of a thrombus in the coronary arteries. Sudden death had followed a severe paroxysm with well-defined softening of the heart muscle.'

But then, in the early decades of the twentieth century, the nature of this strongly age-determined disease changed dramatically. For no apparent reason it began to afflict otherwise seemingly healthy middle-aged men, increasing year on year to become much the commonest cause of premature death. The cause of this 'epidemic' remained obscure but from the 1980s onwards, Professor Geoffrey Rose and his fellow epidemiologists would assert with increasing conviction the culprit to be those 'high fat' foods in raising the cholesterol level in the blood. The wide acceptance of this 'diet-heart thesis', as it became known, would pave the way for the mass prescription of cholesterol-lowering statins. It is not possible to comprehend how this came about without an historical perspective on 'The Rise and Fall of Heart Disease'.

Chapter 3

The Rise and Fall of Heart Disease

The modern epidemic of heart disease started quite suddenly in the 1930s. Doctors had no difficulty in recognising its gravity because so many of their colleagues were among its early victims, apparently healthy middle-aged physicians who, for no obvious reason, suddenly collapsed and died. Within a decade, heart disease had become much the commonest cause of death in the weekly obituary columns of the medical journals. This new disease clearly required a name. The cause, it seemed, was a clot of blood (or thrombus) in the arteries to the heart, which had been narrowed by a porridge-like substance, atheroma, made up of fibrous material and a type of fat called cholesterol. These are the 'coronary' arteries, for they form a 'crown' or corona at the top of the heart before passing over its surface to provide oxygenated blood to the heart muscle. Hence the blockage of one or other of these arteries with a thrombus became known as a 'coronary thrombosis' or simply 'a coronary', better known as a 'heart attack'.

The novelty of this epidemic of coronary disease was emphasised in 1946 by Sir Maurice Cassidy, the king's physician,
in the prestigious Harveian Oration. He first noted that the
numbers dying from heart disease had increased ten-fold in
just over a decade, and then confirmed that, from his own
clinical experience, 'coronary thrombosis is far more prevalent than it was. Looking through my notes of patients seen
twenty or more years ago, I come across occasional cases where
I failed to recognise it, which now appeared to be the obvious
diagnosis, but such cases are exceptionally few.' And what
possibly could be the reason why apparently fit and healthy
men in their forties and fifties should suddenly have their
lives snuffed out in this way? Sir Maurice was puzzled. The
presence of atheroma in the coronary arteries that appeared
to predispose to a heart attack is almost universal, certainly in
the elderly in Western societies, so one would naturally expect
coronary thrombosis to have been a common disease in the
past. On the contrary, the first description in Britain of the
characteristic severe crushing chest pain followed by sudden
death of a heart attack in middle-aged men had been reported
just twenty years earlier in 1925: 'In sudden thrombosis of the
coronary arteries, there may occur a very characteristic clinical
syndrome which has attracted little attention in Britain and
which receives scant attention in the text books.' It seemed to
Sir Maurice that the key to the epidemic must lie in the clot or
thrombus, but what precipitated it, he admitted, 'is a problem
I have failed to solve'.

Among those interested in 'solving the problem' was
Ancel Keys, the forty-year-old Director of the Laboratory of
Physiological Hygiene at the University of Minnesota, who at
the close of the war turned his attention to investigating why so

many middle-aged men were dying from heart attacks. His particular scientific interest was nutrition, and so naturally enough he focused his attention on the fat chemical cholesterol present in the atheroma of the arteries. The main source of cholesterol is the liver, from where it is released into the bloodstream to fulfil its indispensable role as an integral component of the cells of the body, as well as being the precursor of many important hormones, including testosterone in the male and oestrogen in the female. Perhaps, Keys speculated, cholesterol-rich foods such as eggs and avocados might, in combination with meat and dairy products that are high in 'saturated fat', force up the level of cholesterol in the blood, which would then infiltrate the artery walls to form the atheroma that appeared to be implicated in heart attacks. It was not an original idea, but Ancel Keys was to pursue it so vigorously over the coming years as essentially to make it his own.

First, it was necessary to know more about the predisposing or 'risk factors' for a coronary, so Keys set up a study, involving almost 300 businessmen from his home town of Minneapolis. They were weighed and measured, their cholesterol levels monitored, their blood pressure recorded and their fate followed over the succeeding twenty-five years. From this it emerged that three main 'risk factors' – smoking (of course), raised blood pressure and a high cholesterol level – together markedly increased the subsequent risk of a coronary. There was, however, a problem. The implication of food consumption in the heart disease epidemic would have been straightforward had the Minnesota businessmen with high cholesterol levels been at 'greater risk' because they consumed more saturated fat. But this was not the case. Their diet was no different from those with normal or even low cholesterol levels.

It remained a puzzle until, almost inadvertently, Keys stumbled on what he believed must be the answer while on a trip to Rome in 1951 to chair a United Nations committee. The professor of physiology at the University of Naples pointed out that heart disease was 'not a problem' in his city. He invited Keys to come and see for himself, and the following year Keys and his wife Margaret, a trained biochemist who specialised in measuring cholesterol levels in the blood, arrived in Naples. They set up their cholesterol-measuring equipment and soon their Neapolitan friends were bringing in workers from the neighbourhood. Their cholesterol levels turned out to be one-third lower than those of the businessmen they had been studying back in Minnesota. The explanation for why heart disease was 'not a problem' in Naples had to be the Neapolitan diet:

'There is no mistaking the general picture – a little lean meat once or twice a week was the rule, butter was almost unknown, milk was never drunk except in coffee or for infants, "colazione" on the job often meant half a loaf of bread crammed with baked lettuce or spinach. Pasta was eaten every day, usually also with bread (no spreads) and a fourth of the calories were provided by olive oil and wine.'

Over the next few years Keys travelled the world investigating the relationship between diet and coronary heart disease in different countries, culminating in 1956 with visits in the same year to the city of Fukuoka in Japan and the province of North Karelia in Finland. The Japanese famously enjoy fish, rice and pickled foods with little meat and few dairy products, and the blood samples taken from Japanese farmers, clerks and coal miners revealed – by now predictably enough – a low cholesterol level in the blood. Meanwhile the eminent cardiologist Paul White, accompanying them, 'spent weeks trying to find a single case of coronary thrombosis in the big medical school hospital, district hospitals and private clinics'.

Later the same year Keys arrived with his entourage in North Karelia, on the Finnish border with Russia – where the pattern of food consumption could scarcely have been more different:

'The first village they visited had an infirmary with six beds for male patients. One was a young man who had been bitten by a bear. A second had cancer of the lung and the third was occupied by an old man wheezing with asthma. The other three patients had coronary heart disease. Later we went into the woods to have a sauna with some lumberjacks. Two of them confessed to being slowed up by angina, but even more interesting was a glimpse into the local eating habits, the favoured "after-sauna" snack was a slab of full-fat cheese the size of a slice of bread on which was smeared a thick layer of "that good Finnish butter".'

Ancel Keys's findings became more persuasive still when he combined them. As clearly demonstrated in Figure 3.1, there appears to be a direct correlation between the amount of saturated fat in a nation's diet and the prevalence of heart disease – with Japan in the bottom left-hand corner, Finland in the top right-hand corner and the United States and Italy in between. What more evidence could one need?

There remained the possibility that the marked difference in susceptibility to heart disease might be due to genetic differences. Keys tackled the question in a typically ingenious way. In the 1950s Japan's economy was still devastated by the effects of

Figure 3.1 The number of deaths from heart disease is seven times higher in East Finland compared to Japan and is strongly correlated with the amount of saturated fat (as a proportion of total calories) in the diet

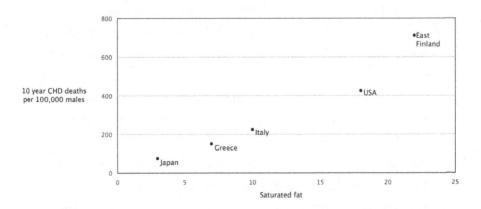

the Second World War, encouraging many Japanese to migrate first to Hawaii – a sort of cultural halfway house – and then to Los Angeles. Keys examined the coronary mortality rates among Japanese migrants to Hawaii and Los Angeles and compared the figures with those obtained from the indigenous Japanese of Fukuoka. There was a clear gradient: as the Japanese became progressively more westernised, so their cholesterol levels rose. As Keys put it, 'the conclusion seemed to be inescapable – the proportion of calories provided by saturated fat (meat, milk and dairy products) is an important factor in the frequency of coronary heart disease' (see Figure 3.2). Thus was born the 'diet-heart thesis', the solution to the problem that Sir Maurice Cassidy had admitted ten years previously 'I cannot solve': too much fat in the diet pushes up the cholesterol level in the blood, which infiltrates and narrows the walls of the coronary arteries, resulting in a heart attack.

Figure 3.2 The rate of heart disease in Japanese migrants increases when they adopt a 'high fat' Western diet

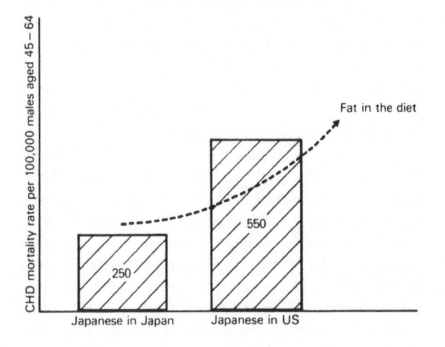

By the mid-1950s, Ancel Keys had become convinced, with good reason, that his original hypothesis – that the epidemic of coronary heart disease was 'a nutritional disorder' caused by 'high fat' foods – must be correct. But when, in 1957, the American Heart Association (AHA) invited a group of heart specialists to evaluate his theory they were unable to endorse it. They noted that despite the impressive differences in rates of heart disease between Japan and Finland, within each country an individual's food preferences neither predicted the level of cholesterol in their blood nor their subsequent risk of heart disease; hence 'high fat' foods could scarcely be a determinant factor. They then turned to two major weaknesses of Keys's

63

theory. First, it failed to account for the very striking 'epidemic' pattern of heart disease noted in Chapter 1 (see Figure 1.2), increasing exponentially year by year from the 1920s to become, by the early 1950s, much the commonest cause of death in middle-aged men. This would have required, if Keys were correct, a sudden dramatic change in the pattern of food consumption in the early decades of the twentieth century, with a sustained increase in the amount of meat, milk and dairy foods consumed. This clearly had not happened.

Next, the Japanese are not the only migrants in the United States. And while the difference in prevalence of heart disease (rare among Japanese in Japan, common among Japanese in Los Angeles) is certainly suggestive of a dietary cause, precisely the same phenomenon can be observed in Swedish migrants. Swedes in Sweden have a similar dietary pattern to Americans but with half the rate of heart disease. Yet even though their dietary pattern remains unchanged on moving to the United States, their rate of heart disease doubles (Fig. 3.3). This would suggest that Keys's inference from his Japanese migrant studies reflected a generalised phenomenon whereby migrants from any country would tend to acquire the pattern of disease of their adopted country – which could be for any number of reasons.

Finally, Keys had failed to account for the central feature of a coronary thrombosis – the clot or thrombus in the coronary artery that, by blocking the blood supply to the heart muscle, causes the sudden, dramatic symptoms of a heart attack. As one of his critics, Sir George Pickering, Regius Professor of Medicine at Oxford, was subsequently to observe: '[Keys's thesis] assigns a minor role, in fact almost an afterthought, to the event that determines life or death.'

Figure 3.3 The rate of heart disease in Swedish migrants to the United States almost doubles even though the amount of fat in their diet remains the same

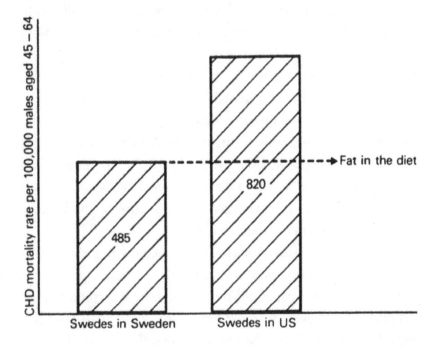

These reservations all pointed to a rather different interpretation of Keys's findings: a 'high fat' diet, along with smoking and raised blood pressure, might be a *contributory* but cannot be a *determinant* factor in the rise of heart disease. The Western diet certainly seemed to explain the higher average cholesterol levels in the West compared to other countries such as Japan, which in turn might predispose individuals to both the narrowed arteries and the clot or thrombus. Moreover, within Western societies, individuals with a genetic predisposition to a higher cholesterol level, such as the Minnesota businessmen, would be at increased risk. But diet could not begin to explain the dramatic rise in incidence of heart disease over the previous fifty years without a truly monumental increase in the amount of meat and dairy products consumed. Keys was half right – heart disease does have 'something to do with' cholesterol levels. But, from the important point of view of preventing heart disease, it was, regrettably, the wrong half. It would be quite unrealistic to expect people to make the major changes required in switching from a Western-style to a Mediterranean- or Japanese-style diet, when the resultant fall in cholesterol would only indirectly reduce the risk of a heart attack. A subtle point, perhaps, but sometimes subtlety can be important. And so, the American Heart Association committee concluded, 'The evidence does not convey any specific implications for drastic dietary changes.'

The verdict was a serious blow. It conveyed the impression that Keys's scientific work over the previous ten years, impressive as it undoubtedly was, could not sustain the interpretation he had placed on it. Keys was just one of many scientists who had backed the wrong horse. Nor was he the only person to be discomfited. The careers of several other scientists who had rallied to his banner would similarly founder in the absence of official endorsement. The most prominent of these, and destined to become Keys's lifelong friend, was Jeremiah Stamler of Chicago University. In 1957, at the time of the publication of the AHA report, Stamler was about to launch the Coronary Prevention Evaluation Program, whose purpose, as its name implies, was to demonstrate that heart disease was indeed preventable by encouraging people to take more exercise, stop smoking and change to a 'healthy' (low fat) diet. The AHA's failure to endorse the need for 'drastic dietary change' placed him in the same invidious position as Keys – vulnerable to the charge of dietary crankery, someone whose ideas were outside the mainstream of medical thinking.

Clearly the American Heart Association had to be persuaded to change its mind. It took some time, but within a couple of years membership of the relevant committee had been reconstituted to include both Keys and Stamler. Its next report, predictably, was very different in tone and content from the first, running to a mere two pages, thus omitting any discussion of the substantial problems of Keys's thesis. Reversing the previous conclusion, it recommended that people should indeed reduce the amount of fat in their diet in anticipation of reducing the risk of heart disease while admitting there was, as yet, 'no final proof'. This might seem a trivial matter but, as would be seen, it would profoundly influence public beliefs, government policy and the practice of medicine for the next four decades.

Keys and Stamler then had a stroke of luck. The main contending explanation of heart disease – that the most important factor was the clot or thrombus in the coronary artery – collapsed with the publication in 1964 of an authoritative study evaluating the benefits of blood-thinning drugs (anticoagulants), which should, if the clot was the critical factor, have had a major impact on the risk of a heart attack. These drugs, it emerged, could indeed reduce the risk of a heart attack by 'thinning' the blood, but this benefit was balanced by an increase in the numbers in whom the anticoagulants had also resulted – as they were likely to – in causing a fatal haemorrhage into the brain.

It was at this crucial moment that Keys's thesis emerged, now endorsed (thanks to his efforts) by the AHA and without a serious challenger, to become the central explanation of the coronary epidemic – an epidemic now so severe that virtually any explanation would have served as a way to make sense of why for over thirty years the toll of predominantly middle-aged men dying from coronaries had increased exponentially year by year, with absolutely no sign of it coming to an end.

The imagery invoked was certainly (and remains) very powerful – indeed it might seem self-evident that those foolish enough to indulge in a cooked breakfast of bacon and eggs should, by pushing up the cholesterol levels in their blood, increase their chances of keeling over with a coronary. The proposed solution of embracing a more ascetic lifestyle seemed similarly plausible, and was certainly consistent with the increasingly influential notion that an 'unhealthy' Western diet not only lay behind the epidemic of heart disease but was also responsible for other common illnesses such as stroke and cancer. Whereas poverty had been a major factor in illness in the past, with increasing prosperity the Western world was now plagued with these 'diseases of affluence'. Or, as the Assistant Secretary of Health to the United States Government informed a Congress sub-committee, 'While scientists do not yet agree on the specific causal relationships, there is a general agreement that the kinds and amounts of food we consume in our affluent societies may be the major factor associated with causes of cancer, circulatory disorders and other chronic illnesses.'

Still the evidence remained circumstantial. There was as yet no incontrovertible proof that a combination of dietary changes to lower the cholesterol level with modifications of the other risk factors could prevent the tragedy of all those tens of thousands of premature deaths. To this end the protagonists in both the United States and Europe launched, in the early 1970s, the largest and most expensive scientific experiment ever conceived in the history of medicine, involving over 60,000 men and costing in excess of £100 million.

In the United States, 360,000 middle-aged men were interviewed to find the 12,000 at highest risk. Most were smokers, had been diagnosed as having raised blood pressure while still young and had markedly elevated cholesterol levels. They were then randomly allocated into either an 'intervention' or a 'control' group, and the Multiple Risk Factor Intervention Trial (MRFIT) was launched. The complexity and expense of this study lay in the need to change people's lives – to encourage them to give up one style of life and adopt another. There was little difficulty in ensuring that those with raised blood pressure were adequately treated by giving appropriate medication. Discouraging smoking was, as always, more difficult, and every conceivable way was deployed to encourage the men to quit, including monetary rewards, hypnosis and aversion techniques. But such practicalities were nothing when compared to what was required to achieve the dietary modifications necessary to lower the cholesterol level. Nothing other than monumental changes would do, so the participants were showered with nutritional information, taught how to shop for groceries and what to order in restaurants, given advice on how to rewrite their favourite recipes, asked to record everything they ate and sign contracts pledging to abstain from various foods. They were told to buy only low fat milk and dairy products, restricted to two eggs a week and instructed to markedly reduce the amount of meat consumed. These prodigious efforts were rewarded: the average amount of saturated fat in their diet fell by about a quarter, but disappointingly their cholesterol level fell only by just over 5 per cent.

The dedication and energy of those involved in the MRFIT trial was admirable, but it would be quite unrealistic to expect that such prodigious efforts would be readily applicable in the real world. Hence the interest in the second of the two studies launched at the same time and organised by the already encountered Geoffrey Rose, Professor of Epidemiology at the London School of Hygiene and the leading standard-bearer for Keys's hypothesis in Europe. His project, co-ordinated under the auspices of the World Health Organisation and thus known as the WHO trial, was four times larger, involving almost 50,000 men in sixty-six factories in Britain, Belgium, Italy and Poland. The workers in the 'intervention' group were exposed to a blitzkrieg of health education to encourage them to change their lifestyle, backed up by evening meetings, talks about heart disease and cookery demonstrations. Those in the 'control' factories were left in peace.

It would seem unlikely, given how the rise in heart disease could not be explained by increasing amounts of saturated fat in the diet, that these radical dietary changes to reduce fat consumption would be effective in preventing it. And so it turned out. Despite the prodigious efforts of the MRFIT trial to cajole so many men into changing their lives and giving up the pleasures of meat, eggs and much else besides, the results published in 1982 revealed they were no less likely to suffer from a heart attack than those in the 'control' group. Seven months later the WHO trial delivered precisely the same verdict.

Thus, the diet-heart thesis had been put to the test in two quite different ways. The first, as represented by the trials, was to encourage people to change their diets and see the effect on heart disease. This, as has been noted, had no effect. The second was to perform the experiment, as it were, the other way round, examining whether the dramatic increased incidence in heart disease over the previous decades had been paralleled by major changes in what people ate. This, as has also already been noted, had always been a central weakness of the thesis, as the twenty-fold rise in heart disease through the 1940s and 1950s had not been paralleled by increasing amounts of meat and dairy products in the diet. Then, suddenly and inexplicably, in the mid-1960s, the remorseless upward trend reversed – already so vividly portrayed in the graph of the changing pattern of heart disease in the United States (see again Figure 1.2) – and the incidence of heart disease went into steep decline. The decline, it must be appreciated, was universal, across all ages, classes and ethnic groups, and international, occurring simultaneously first in the United States, Canada, New Zealand and Australia, and followed a decade later by Britain and the countries of Western Europe. Thus, if the 'lifestyle' theory of heart disease were correct, people must have made substantial changes in their diet at least ten years earlier, not just in the United States but in all these other countries as well. Clearly, this was impossible, for (as shown in Figure 3.4) the precipitous rise and equally precipitous fall in heart disease occurs in different countries in parallel, while the total amount of fat in the diet hardly changes. Indeed, by the early 1980s, as the fall in heart disease accelerated it became obvious that, were diet a major factor through its effect on cholesterol levels, there would have to have been monumental changes – much greater than those imposed on the 'intervention' group in the MRFIT trial. Rather, this pattern of a 'rise and fall' of heart disease is scarcely compatible with it being due primarily to social factors such as an individual's food preferences; instead it strongly resembles the 'rise and fall' of an infectious epidemic. Perhaps, then, some unknown biological agent might be the primary cause, either by influencing the severity of atheroma in the coronary arteries or precipitating the clot that caused the heart attack, or both.

Figure 3.4 The precipitous rise and fall in heart disease occurs in several countries in parallel while the total amount of fat in the diet remains stable

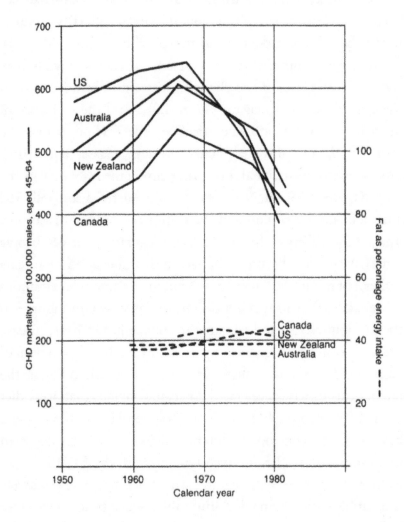

The seriousness of these developments for the proponents of the diet-heart thesis is obvious enough. They were just getting into their stride with their ambitious programme to realign medicine towards preventing the diseases of affluence

and now suddenly the scientific validity of its central pillar – the implication of the Western diet in the epidemic of heart disease – seemed highly questionable. Two powerful interested parties could not acknowledge defeat. The first were the nutritionists and epidemiologists like Keys, Stamler, Rose and many others who had invested a lifetime's work and hundreds of millions in research funds in trying to prove the thesis. The second were the drug companies who had invested heavily in the development of cholesterol-lowering drugs for which, naturally, they needed a market. Now cholesterol, as has been noted, is not entirely innocent: whatever unknown 'biological' cause might account for that striking pattern of the 'rise and fall' of heart disease, it is more likely to affect those with higher than average cholesterol levels, and therefore more severe atheroma in their coronary arteries. Hence, both the dietary protagonists and the drug companies had a mutual interest in salvaging the diet-heart thesis. If the drug companies could show their powerful cholesterol-lowering drugs reduced the chances of a heart attack in those with markedly raised cholesterol levels (which was probable), this would be evidence the disease was indeed 'preventable' – which would then shore up the position of the proponents of the dietary theory like Keys and Rose. If they could, in their turn, convince the public that too much meat, milk and cheese caused heart disease, so everyone should lower their cholesterol levels, this would markedly increase the market for cholesterol-lowering drugs way beyond the minority 'at high risk'. And that is precisely what happened.

We start with the dietary protagonists. Clearly, if the diet-heart thesis were to be salvaged, despite the negative results of the trials, the focus would have to be shifted away from the scientific arena where it could be debated towards authoritative *ex cathedra* assertions that bacon and eggs (or their equivalent) really did cause heart attacks. The best way of ensuring this 'fact management' was through the medium of reports from 'expert committees' made up of the protagonists – the same ploy by which Ancel Keys had persuaded the American Heart Association to endorse his thesis back in 1961. From 1982 to 1987 seven different reports came to precisely the same verdict, that the Western diet caused heart disease (and strokes and breast cancer and much else besides), and argued for major changes in the nation's diet along the same lines as the MRFIT trial. The consumption of those incriminated 'high fat' foods would have to fall by one-third – rationing meat to a few meals per week, replacing whole milk with skimmed, avoiding 'high fat' cheeses like cheddar and camembert, abjuring butter and treating with caution many highly esteemed foods, from salami to pastries. The omission from these reports of any explanation as to why the definitive trials of this 'healthy' diet in preventing heart disease had proved so unsuccessful prompted a caustic response from the editor of the *International Journal of Cardiology*, Professor J. R. A. Mitchell:

'To those who keep saying that "better eating prevents heart disease" we must reply that every evangelist is entitled to his opinion, but every scientist is entitled to ask for the evidence. The claim that the collective beliefs of a prestigious committee can provide a substitute for facts is all too prevalent ... we can never be sure of the relationship between the opinions of a committee and the truth.'

For all that, each report naturally attracted considerable publicity, and the constant reiteration of a simple message like the drip of water on a stone could not fail to penetrate the public consciousness. Thus, in 1985, the readers of *The Times* were informed: 'Western food is the main single underlying cause of Western disease which leaders of the medical profession [describe] in apocalyptic terms as a holocaust, which medicine can do nothing to check.'

The protagonists were not content to let it rest there. They moved out of their committee rooms into the television studios to hammer the message home. In just two years the BBC and commercial stations launched four separate series promoting the now customary message on diet and disease, each replete with images of food and death that again omitted any allusion to the scientific experiments in which the value of the proposed dietary changes had been assessed.

Opening with a shot of an ambulance screeching through the night or, more gruesomely, a pathologist laying out his tools for a post-mortem, a voiceover intoned chilling statistics about how many people die from certain diseases every year. Then one of the experts would appear to link these diseases to food. Thus Professor Geoffrey Rose: 'The modern British diet is killing people in their thousands from heart attacks.' There was every so often a note of caution, as with Sir Richard Doll: 'There is very little hard evidence but a reasonable estimate would be that diet is responsible for about perhaps one-third of all fatal cancers.' There followed a brief visit to a family that had changed over to the new 'healthy' low fat diet, and concluding remarks against the backdrop of a cemetery. Geoffrey Rose again: 'Behind each one of these statistics is a personal tragedy, each one has left a home with an empty family, without a bread-winner, a wife without a husband, children without supportive parents. We know enough about the causes of these tragedies and their relation to what we eat – if we could get the scientific information across to the public then many of these tragedies would be avoided.'

This very serious state of affairs naturally raised the important question of why so little was being done about it. Every good story requires a villain and, sure enough, the best intentions of the experts were being thwarted by powerful antagonistic forces in the form of the food industry and farmers – and their apologists, a small group of 'corrupt' scientists. 'There are some who, from a position of authority, assert the fat and salt in the quantities consumed in Britain today are harmless to health. As far as I know they are all employed, paid by or associated with the food industry.' The role of these scientific sceptics in condoning the food industry's attempts to peddle lethal foodstuffs to the public was 'the biggest scandal since the day 150 years ago when officials refused to act on the fact that cholera was caused by open sewers'.

As for the second interested party, the pharmaceutical industry, the prospects for the mass prescription of cholesterol-lowering drugs came much closer with the publication in 1984 of a clinical trial demonstrating that, for those with markedly raised cholesterol levels, the drug cholestyramine reduced the chances of a fatal heart attack by 20 per cent. This result, according to the chief organiser, offered 'conclusive proof' that heart disease could be prevented. Admittedly the participants had all been at 'very high risk', but 'the trial's implications could and should be extended to all age groups and those with more modest elevations of cholesterol'.

The following week, the cover of *Time* magazine featured a plate of bacon and eggs arranged to resemble a doleful face with the headline 'CHOLESTEROL: AND NOW THE BAD NEWS ...' 'Sorry, it's true, cholesterol really is a killer,' ran the story on the inside page. *Newsweek* pursued the same line, quoting an expert opinion that this was 'a milestone, with implications for everyone'.

And exactly how did the participants in this 'landmark study' fare? Cholestyramine is not a pill in the conventional sense, but rather comes as a sachet of granules that lowers the cholesterol level by preventing the reabsorption of cholesterol-rich bile acids in the gut. It is not pleasant to take, rendering food unpalatable and irritating the lining of the gut, with two-thirds of the participants reporting moderate to serious side effects of constipation, gas, heartburn and bloating. Still, such misfortunes might be endured if cholestyramine really did reduce one's chances of a fatal heart attack by such a substantial margin as 20 per cent. The future, after all, is an unknown territory and many in their forties and beyond, conscious of their inevitable mortality, might think it merely perverse not to ensure that it be later rather than sooner, preventing – or at least postponing – the inevitable.

This brings us to the sleight of hand, alluded to in the previous chapter, that sustains the vast edifice of mass medicalisation, portraying drugs as being vastly more advantageous than they really are. To appreciate how it works, we have to pay attention to the small print. We start with Table 3.1 and contrast the first and second rows. The first row gives us a 'relative risk' reduction of cardiac events (that is heart attacks) and cardiac deaths, with a 'relative' reduction of respectively 20 per cent and 25 per cent – hence the claim that cholestyramine reduces the risks of a fatal heart attack by a quarter. The second row seems much less impressive; here the 'absolute risk reduction' for any individual is just 0.4 per cent, i.e. only 0.4 per cent of participants benefit by not having a fatal heart attack. Whence comes the discrepancy between these figures?

Table 3.1 The striking difference between the 'relative' and 'absolute' benefits of cholestyramine in reducing the risk of heart attacks and coronary deaths

	Cardiac events	Cardiac deaths
Relative rate reduction	−20%	−20%
Absolute rate reduction	−1.8%	−0.4%

Now we must turn to Table 3.2, which gives us the numbers – 155 cardiac events in those taking cholestyramine compared to 187 in those with a placebo, i.e. 32 fewer, which seems very useful. But if you look at the number of people suffering a cardiac event as a percentage of all those in the trial, this works out at respectively 8.1 per cent and 9.8 per cent. Repeating the exercise for cardiac deaths, there are eight fewer in the cholestyramine group compared to the placebo group; the percentage of each group that had a fatal heart attack is respectively 1.6 per cent and 2.0 per cent.

Table 3.2 The results of the cholestyramine trial

	Placebo (n=1900)	Rate %	Cholestyramine (n=1906)	Rate %
Cardiac events	187	9.8	155	8.1
Cardiac mortality	38	2.0	30	1.6
Deaths from all causes	71	3.7	68	3.6

And now for the sting. One can indeed claim 20 per cent fewer cardiac events in those taking cholestyramine, as 9.8 (placebo) minus 8.1 (cholestyramine) gives us 1.7, which is roughly one-fifth (or 20 per cent) of the placebo figure. That is, 'relative' to the numbers in the placebo group there are 20 per cent fewer cardiac events in those taking cholestyramine. But in absolute terms, the benefit for the individual is just 1.7 per cent, that is just 1.7 out of 100 of those taking cholestyramine will benefit. And repeating the exercise for cardiac deaths, there are indeed 20 per cent fewer in those taking cholestyramine, because the difference between 2.0 (placebo) and 1.6 (cholestyramine) of 0.4 is roughly 20 per cent of the placebo figure. But, again, in absolute terms it reduces the individual's chance of dying from a coronary by just 0.4 per cent. Or, put another way, just 1 in 250 of those taking cholestyramine benefited by having their 'life saved', compared to the 249 who did not. Again, one might wonder who would willingly take cholestyramine for seven years on the off-chance they would be the lucky person out of so many whose life might be saved by doing so. And that is how, as noted in the Introduction, the drug companies systematically exaggerate the benefits of their drugs, here by fifty-fold (20 being 50 times greater than 0.4).

Still, this is not quite the last word. The bottom line of Table 3.2 gives the total numbers of people dying during the trial in both groups. Here, we note, there is virtually no difference – 71 (3.7 per cent) of those taking the placebo compared to 68 (3.6 per cent) of those taking cholestyramine – the modest reduction in 'cardiac deaths' being balanced by an increased risk of dying from 'other causes'. The upshot of all this is that while the organisers of the trial were indeed correct in claiming that cholestyramine reduced the (relative) risk of a fatal coronary by 20 per cent, they could, had they so wished, have presented a more balanced evaluation of its merits, at least from the patient's perspective, that this means just one life saved for every 250 people taking the drug. They might also, had they so wished, have pointed out that seven years' worth of cholestyramine for the 1906 men in the trial cost £9 million, which works out at over £1 million for each of the eight fatal heart attacks prevented. And, as there was no significant difference in overall mortality, an infinite sum for every life saved.

Still, this was the first 'definitive proof' of the merits of cholesterol lowering. And, with the imminent prospect of further, much better tolerated drugs, the next task was to raise the public's consciousness about their life-saving potential. Now for a further sting. It is only natural to be a bit suspicious when a drug company extols the benefits of its new wonder drug X, but an entirely different matter when the desirability of taking such a drug is endorsed by independent experts as part of an 'education' programme. And sure enough, in December 1984, just a few months after the cholestyramine trial, the US National Institute of Health launched the National Cholesterol Education Program with the double message: 'The blood cholesterol level of most Americans is undesirably high' and it should be reduced because 'it has been established beyond reasonable doubt' that this will reduce the subsequent risk of a heart attack. The programme started by reasserting the fundamental message of the diet-heart thesis – everyone should make substantial reductions in the amount of meat, milk and dairy products they consume so as to reduce the amount of fat in their diet by a quarter. Next, people needed to know their 'number' (i.e. their cholesterol level) – and the tens of millions in whom it was higher than 'normal' (i.e. the half of the population in whom it was greater than the average of 5 millimoles per litre) would then require dietary advice to lower it. This, unless vigorously adhered to, did not work – leaving no option other than the prescription of cholesterol-lowering drugs.

Thus, the ground was well and truly prepared when, in 1987, the drug company Merck launched its new drug lovastatin (under the name Mevacor), the first of the statins – which, being so much better tolerated than cholestyramine, would eventually, when taken by millions, generate the greatest financial bonanza in the history of the pharmaceutical industry. The National Cholesterol Education Program thus proved very useful to the drug companies. The suspicion that its seemingly authoritative advice was not quite as dispassionate as it might have been seems to be confirmed by Merck's press release announcing the launch of lovastatin, which included the names and telephone numbers of doctors that journalists could contact for their comments on the benefits of this new wonder drug. They included Scott M. Grundy, the chairman of the committee drawing up the Education Program's recommendations, Daniel Steinberg, the physician who had developed the details of the programme, and Antonio Gott, no less than the President of the American Heart Association itself.

The strategy worked brilliantly. The fear of premature death from a coronary was quite sufficient to propel the health-conscious to their doctor's surgery to have their cholesterol level measured and 'learn their number'; a quarter of whom would subsequently be started on drug therapy.

Together the proponents of dietary change and the drug companies had triumphed. Snatching victory from the jaws of defeat, dozens of expert committee reports would persuade most people that 'Western food is the chief reason for our modern epidemic of heart disease'. This in turn would be the stalking horse by which drug companies would persuade millions that they needed to take their cholesterol-lowering statins for life. They are, as will be seen, vastly less efficacious than commonly perceived – inevitably so, for cholesterol can only be a subsidiary contributory factor to that dramatic rise and fall in heart disease over the past century. This will become readily apparent in the epilogue to this chapter.

* * *

Epilogue: The causes of coronary heart disease

Coronary heart disease, along with strokes and cancer, is age-determined. The longer you live, the greater the risk – one which increases exponentially decade by decade as the walls of the arteries, buffeted by the blood pumping through the circulation, become progressively hardened and narrowed. In Western society, then, it is a 'natural event', one that may be postponed but is no more truly preventable than ageing itself.

But the cause of that dramatic rise and fall in the incidence of heart disease in predominantly middle-aged men over the past seventy years remains unknown. This is not in itself surprising for despite the many achievements of medicine, the causes of the vast majority of illnesses similarly remain unknown – that is, virtually all the neurological disorders such as multiple sclerosis, the rheumatological disorders such as rheumatoid arthritis, the dermatological disorders such as psoriasis, the gut disorders such as Crohn's disease, and so on. To be sure, factors such as cigarette smoking, markedly raised cholesterol and a genetic predisposition will increase the risk, making a coronary more probable. But they do not distinguish between those who might or might not sustain one.

Rather the striking pattern of the rise and fall is strongly suggestive of an infectious epidemic and indeed the state of the lining of the arteries narrowed by atherosclerosis, when examined under the microscope, resembles an inflammatory process such as might be caused by a virus or bacterium. The specific culprit, however, remains elusive. In 1992, Dr Chochuo Kuo of the University of Washington identified the bacterium chlamydia in the walls of the arteries of South African miners who had recently succumbed to a heart attack. This prompted several studies looking for further evidence of chronic infection that would implicate variously the bacterium mycoplasma and viruses including herpes and cytomegalovirus. Dr Stephen Epstein, also of the University of Washington, observes in reflecting on these findings:

'Compelling evidence has accrued suggesting that certain infectious agents contribute to the cause of atherosclerosis. It is clear, however, that the relationship is extremely complex ... It is the aggregate number of certain bacteria rather than any specific infectious agent that determines the propensity to develop atherosclerosis and the acute [coronary event].'

This is no mere conjecture, for there is a compelling parallel with another illness, peptic ulcer of the stomach, that has exhibited a similar dramatic 'rise and fall' pattern over the past one hundred years, attributed to increased acidic secretions from, variously, stress, an anxious personality and eating the wrong type of food. Then in 1983 a young Australian doctor Barry Marshall identified a novel type of bacterium (helicobacter) in the lining of the stomach whose role in causing those peptic ulcers provided a coherent explanation while opening up the possibility of a genuinely effective treatment with antibiotics.

Thus a nuanced view of the causes of heart disease would take into account several considerations. First, like stroke and most cancer, it is age determined – the longer you live the greater the risk of a heart attack or fatal coronary, three quarters of which occur in those aged seventy and beyond. Superimposed on this the striking pattern of that rise and fall affecting mostly middle-aged men is strongly suggestive of an unknown (though probably infectious) biological cause with an increased risk in smokers and those with a raised cholesterol. But nuance does not sell drugs and we turn now to consider how cholesterol-lowering drugs would become the biggest the money spinner of all.

Chapter 4

All Must Take Statins

In 1976 Henry Gadsden, brilliant chairman of (at the time) the world's most profitable and innovative drug company, Merck, expressed disappointment that the potential market for his company's drugs was limited to treating only the sick. His vision, he told an interviewer for *Forbes* magazine, was rather that they should be making drugs for the healthy as well, for then they could 'sell to everyone' – in the same way that Wrigley's marketed their chewing gum. He was only half joking. His vision, an inspired strategic response to the recent downturn in the pharmaceutical industry's fortunes, proved remarkably prescient. Forty years later Merck's revenues, along with those of all the other major drug companies, would have increased forty-fold, making pharmaceuticals by far the world's most profitable industry. This is how it happened.

Merck had been in at the beginning of the therapeutic revolution in the mid-1940s that would transform the practice of medicine in the decades after the Second World War. The company played a central role in the assault on infectious disease – first pioneering the mass production of the legendary penicillin and, soon after, discovering streptomycin, the first cure for tuberculosis, till then so aptly described as 'The Captain of the Armies of Death'. Merck was the first too to synthesise cortisone, which would not only prove invaluable in the treatment of more than two hundred previously untreatable conditions, but facilitate the heretofore seemingly inconceivable goals of transplanting hearts and kidneys and curing deadly illnesses such as childhood leukaemia. The vast market for these drugs and the prodigious profits to be made from just one discovery encouraged Merck and all its competitors to invest heavily in research, for which they were richly rewarded with a cornucopia of new drugs that came cascading out of their laboratories. Some idea of the extraordinary scale of this phenomenon can be gleaned from Table 4.1, which charts, decade by decade, the discoveries of that 'golden age', with effective treatments for the entire spectrum of infectious illness, cancer, mental illness (schizophrenia, depression and bipolar disorder), crippling rheumatological disorders, Parkinson's disease, epilepsy, asthma, and much else besides. The vast majority remain in routine use to this day.

But there is a limit to the number of chemicals that might be investigated for their therapeutic potential, and by the early seventies this Golden Age was drawing to a close. There was 'A Dearth of New Drugs', observed the editor of the science journal *Nature*, commenting on a recent analysis showing the number of new drugs each year dropping off sharply from over seventy in the 1960s to less than twenty: 'The identification of many biologically important chemicals after the war may have created a fruitful basis for innovation but has subsequently shown diminishing returns.' Nor was it merely proving harder to come up with genuinely new drugs. An analysis of the most recent introductions found that many seemed to offer only 'moderate therapeutic gain'; in other words they were little better than those already available.

This sharp decline in the numbers of new drugs is most readily attributable to the tightening of regulations following the thalidomide disaster, when thousands of children were born with shortened or absent limbs to mothers prescribed the drug early in pregnancy. In Britain from 1969 onwards, toxicity testing in animals became mandatory, followed by the requirement for several stages of clinical trials in humans before new drugs could be approved. This naturally made the whole process of developing new drugs much more complicated and therefore expensive – unnecessarily so, claimed the pharmaceutical industry. Over-regulation had, it was alleged, if not exactly killed off the golden goose, certainly reduced its production of golden eggs.

But the 'dearth of new drugs' was not just a matter of over-regulation, as evidenced by an ever-widening gap between the scale of investment in research and its returns. This was attributed variously to the notion that the 'easy' therapeutic advances had already been made and to the difficulty of improving on the efficacy of those drugs already discovered. It was one thing for researchers back in the 1940s to have stumbled (for example) on penicillin and other antibiotics effective against the full range of infectious illness, quite another to understand the complexities of diseases like Alzheimer's or multiple sclerosis and find some effective remedies against them. Indeed, the pharmaceutical industry had become in a way a victim of its own success, for the effectiveness of antibiotics like penicillin and streptomycin in

Table 4.1 The Golden Age of drug discovery 1940–1975

	Infections diseases	Cancer	Psychiatry	Rheumatology
1940	Penicillin Streptomycin PAS Chloramphenicol Tetracyline Cephalosporin	Antibiotics Cortisone Methotrexate 6-mp	Lithium	Antibiotics Cortisone Methotrexate
1950	Nystatin Erythromycin Vancomycin Kanamycin Amphotericin B Griseofulvin Metronidazole	Thiothepa Chlorambucil Melphalan Cyclophosphamide Actinomycin 5-FU	Chlorpromazine Imipramine Marsilid Meprobomate Haloperidol	Phenylbutazone Hydroxychloroquine Cyclophosphamide
1960	Fusidic acid Lincomycin Gentamycin Ethambutol Clotrimazole Trimethoprim Rifampicin Amantadine Idoxuridine	Daunomycin Bleomycin L-Asparaginase Vincristine Cisplatin	Diazepam Chlordiazepoxide	Indomethacin Ibuprofen Penicillamine Allopurinol Mefanamic acid
1970	Carbenicillin Interferon		Fluoxetine Clozapine	Diflunisal Piroxicam

All Must Take Statins

Circulatory disorders	Endocrinology	Other: neurology (N), haematology (H), gastroenterology (G), respiratory illness (R)
Lignocaine	Carbimazole	Antibiotics
Hydralazine	Stilboestrol	Cortisone
Acetazolamide	Vasopressin	Vitamin B12 (H)
		Vitamin K (H)
Clofibrate	Chlorpropramide	Bisacodyl (G)
Methyldopa	Phenformin	Factor VIII (H)
Disopyramide	HRT	Primidone (N)
Spironolactone		Ethosuximide (N)
Chlorothiazide		Isoprenaline (R)
Propranolol	The 'Pill'	Azathioprine
Verapamil	Bromocriptine	L-dopa (N)
Frusemide	HCG	Carbamazapine (N)
Chlorestyramine	Clomiphene	Naloxone (N)
Clonidine	Tamoxifen	Sodium valproate (N)
Amiloride		Carbenoxolone (G)
		Salbutamol (R)
		Sodium chromoglycate (R)
		Chlormethiazole (G)
Captopril		Cyclosporin
Nifedipine		Metoclopramide (G)
Amiodarone		Cimetidine (G)
Dipyrimadole		Cheonodeoxycholic acid (G)

curing life-threatening pneumonias or tuberculosis necessarily constrained the potential market for yet another of this class of drugs. Thus, 'If the industry was to have a viable future it would be necessary to grasp the nature of this irony and invert it,' observes Jeremy Greene, Professor of the History of Science at Harvard University. 'Drugs needed to *grow* their market not shrink them.'

And so we return to Henry Gadsden and his unsettling 'solution' to this 'dearth of new drugs' – for certainly the most obvious way to grow the market was to target the millions of the healthy. And the key to that lay in the concept of 'pharmaceutical prevention', the identification among the legions of healthy those with raised blood pressure or cholesterol levels that increased the risk of heart disease and stroke.

It had worked for severe hypertension, as demonstrated by the famous Veterans' trial involving one of Merck's most successful drugs, the antihypertensive chlorothiazide, a drug which proved to be so much more profitable still when prescribed to the vastly greater numbers with 'mild hypertension'. The challenge was to do the same, on a much grander scale, for heart disease. We saw in the previous chapter how, together, the epidemiological evangelists for the diet-heart thesis and the pharmaceutical industry had salvaged victory from the jaws of defeat (the failure of the massive lifestyle intervention trials) to assert the central determinant role of raised cholesterol as a primary cause of the heart disease epidemic – culminating in that cholestyramine trial with its 'definitive proof' of the benefits of lowering cholesterol. But cholestyramine was so unpalatable, its side effects so unpleasant, it was unrealistic to suppose that legions of the healthy could be persuaded to take it indefinitely in anticipation of reducing their risks of a fatal heart attack by (as misleadingly claimed) one-quarter. Rather, the future direction and prosperity of the pharmaceutical industry rested on Merck's more potent and much better tolerated lovastatin, waiting in the wings as it were to begin its dizzying ascent as the first of the most profitable class of drugs ever discovered. Henry Gadsden's prescient anticipation of selling to the healthy was not mere speculation but informed by his realisation at the time of the potential of this 'novel pharmacological compound', recently discovered by ebullient Japanese researcher Akira Endo, inspired by his understanding – paradox of paradoxes – of cholesterol's indispensable role as one of the most important of all the chemicals in the body. Cholesterol is an essential structural component of the membrane that surrounds each of our several trillion cells and of the myelin sheath that allows for the conduction of electrical signals along the nerves. It is the precursor of the sex hormones testosterone, oestrogen and progesterone, of the adrenal hormones aldosterone and cortisol, and of the bile acids that facilitate the absorption of food and vitamins from the gut and necessary too for the synthesis of the bone-building vitamin D.

Cholesterol is very, very important for all forms of life, including the bacteria that cause pneumonia, bronchitis, kidney infections and so on. Akira Endo speculated that antibiotics such as penicillin do their work in destroying those bacteria by blocking their ability to make that very, very important cho-lesterol. And so it turned out. Following a protracted research programme testing six thousand compounds, he found the first statin that interfered with the third step of what is clearly a very complex process (Figure 4.1).

Hearing of Endo's work, Henry Gadsden invited him to visit Merck's research laboratories, and before long his company's

Figure 4.1 Statins block the third step (HMG-CoA reductase) in the synthesis of cholesterol by the liver

2 acetyl-CoA
↓ acetoacetyl

acetoacetyl-CoA
↓ HMG-CoA synthase

HMG-CoA
↓ HMG-CoA redcutase

mevalonate
↓ mevalonate kinase

5-phosphomevalonate
↓ phosphomevalonate kinase

5-pyrophosphate mevalonate
↓ phosphomevalonate kinase

D3-Isopentenyl pyrophosphate
| isopentenyl-pyrophosphate
↓ isomerase (IPP isomerase)

dimethylallyl pyrophosphate
↓ farnesyl-pyrophosphate transferase

geranyl pyrophosphate
↓ farnesyl-pyrophosphate transferase

farnesyl pyrophosphate
↓ squalene synthase

squalene
↓ squalene epoxidase

squalene 2,3-epoxide
↓ oxidosqualene cyclase

lanosterol
| demethylation
| decarboxylation
↓ migration, reduction of double bonds

CHOLESTEROL

chemists had found a similarly effective chemical, which they named lovastatin. Its launch as Mevacor a decade later, as noted in the previous chapter, coincided in suspiciously neat fashion with the campaign sponsored by the National Cholesterol Education Program urging the public to visit their doctor to learn their cholesterol number. This would be a vital element of the company's 'two-pronged marketing strategy', as a senior director explained:

'Our primary effort will be devoted to gaining physician awareness and acceptance of Mevacor as a major break-through in the treatment of elevated cholesterol. At the same time, we will work with various organisations including the American Heart Association and the National Cholesterol Education Program to foster awareness and knowledge of the risks associated with elevated cholesterol.'

The statin era had begun and, just as Gadsden had antici-pated, 'selling to everyone' would salvage the industry's fortunes. Within a couple of years, lovastatin was generating as much rev-enue as Merck's entire drug portfolio had done a decade earlier. Soon, every major drug company would have its own version, and in the fierce competition between them the market would grow a further 25-fold over the next two decades – a process in which the clinical trials necessary to determine their efficacy would play a central role.

This is how it worked. The regulatory process introduced in the aftermath of the thalidomide tragedy required all new drugs to be formally tested for safety and efficacy in clinical trials carried out independently by clinical researchers in teaching hospi-tals and academic centres. This was all straightforward. Thus, investigating the merits of, for example, an anti-inflammatory drug like ibuprofen entailed comparing – in a hundred or so patients – its efficacy against that of a placebo or some similar but different medication. But the process of assessing the merits of cholesterol-lowering drugs is vastly more complex, as here it is necessary to recruit thousands of patients who must then be followed up for several years to see whether there is any difference in, for example, the number of heart attacks in those taking statins against the controls. Such trials can be very costly, to the tune of £100 million or more – and therefore, with so much at stake, drug companies from the 1980s onwards decided to 'take control', as the editor of the *New England Journal of Medicine*, Marcia Angell, describes in a profoundly significant passage in her book *The Truth about the Drug Companies*:

'It used to be that the drug companies simply gave grants to academic medical centres for their researchers to do a study and that was it. The researchers did the study and published the results, whatever they would be. Now it is very, very different. The drug companies increasingly design the studies. They keep the data, they don't even let the researchers see the data. They analyse the data, they decide whether they are going to even publish the data at the end of it. They sign contracts with the researchers and with academic medical centres so that they don't get to publish their work unless they get permission from the drug company. So, you can see that the distortion starts even before publication. It is treating researchers as though they were hired guns, they just do the work. And the drug company will decide what the data shows, what the conclusions are and whether they will even be published.'

In his best-selling critique of the industry, *Bad Pharma*, Ben Goldacre cites fifteen ways ('wily tricks, close calls and elegant mischief at the margins of acceptability') by which drug companies manipulate the data of clinical trials to give the best possible gloss on their findings. Here are three of them:

'*Dodgy sub-group analyses*: If your drug didn't win overall in your trial, you can chop up the data in lots of different ways, to try and see if it won in a sub-group: perhaps it worked brilliantly for Chinese men between the ages of 56 and 71. This is stupid and yet commonplace.

Trials that bundle their outcomes together in odd ways: How you package your data can give misleading results. For example, by setting your thresholds just right, you can turn a modest benefit into an apparently dramatic one. And by bundling up lots of different outcomes to make one big 'composite outcome', you can allow freak results to make it appear that a whole group of outcomes have improved.

Pretend it's all positive regardless: At the end of your trial, if your result is unimpressive, you can exaggerate it in the way that you present the numbers; and if you haven't got a positive result at all, you can just spin harder.'

In this context it is no surprise to learn that the outcome of the twenty-seven major drug company-sponsored statin trials, with the many opportunities for elegant mischief in interpreting their results, proved favourable indeed. Though it would be impossible to consider them in any detail, the verdict is clear enough from examining the two earliest and most influential, which cover the two main indications for statin treatment. The first is for 'primary prevention' in the healthy, to 'primarily' prevent a heart attack, represented here by the West of Scotland Study (WOSCOPS) of 6500 Glaswegian men with raised cholesterol levels. The next is 'secondary' prevention in anticipation of preventing a 'secondary' further episode, represented by the 4S Study in 4444 Swedes with high cholesterol levels and who had already had a heart attack and a history of heart disease.

It helps in appreciating the profound impact these studies had on the rise of mass medicalisation to imagine the situation back in the mid-1990s, where everyone was being vigorously encouraged to 'know their number' and be alert to the mortal dangers of cholesterol, responsible as it was for killing indiscriminately tens of thousands every year. But now it appeared that for many such a fate could be avoided on a spectacular scale. For the healthy (in the WOSCOPS study), taking a statin a day reduced their risk of death from a coronary by one-quarter and for those already with heart disease (the 4S study) by almost a half (40 per cent).

This was clearly a major breakthrough comparable to the cure of tuberculosis or the prevention of polio, or any of the other great triumphs of modern medicine. It made front-page news. Dr Suzanne Oparil, President of the American Heart Association, described the halving of the coronary mortality rate seen in the 4S study as 'dynamite' that 'would change medical practice for ever'. As for the WOSCOPS study, 'For the first time,' wrote health correspondent Jane Brody in the *New York Times*, 'the potent new cholesterol-lowering drugs have been shown to prevent heart attacks in healthy men and women.' Statins were clearly so beneficial that many more of the healthy should benefit from taking them. Soon afterwards, the experts decreed the 'cut-off point' for initiating treatment should be reduced from a cholesterol level of

6.0 to 5.0 – thus, as will be seen (Figure 4.2) from the by now familiar bell curve, increasing the number eligible by almost one-third of the adult population.

Figure 4.2 Reducing the threshold for cholesterol-lowering drugs from 6 to 5 mmol/L markedly increases the numbers eligible for treatment

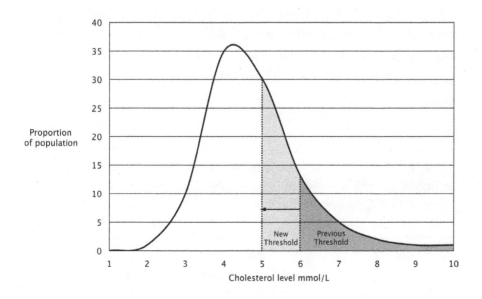

'By the end of the 1990s it had become a commonplace for cardiologists to suggest, only half-jokingly, that statins should be added to the nation's water supply,' noted Professor Jeremy Greene. 'From the pharmaceutical industry's perspective, lowering the threshold for treatment represented a "win-win" arrangement. The lower the threshold, the larger the market, the healthier the pharmaceutical economy. The lower the threshold, the less the mortal and economic cost to the nation from heart disease and stroke. Who could argue against such a convergence of benefit?'

Who indeed? All would welcome the opportunity to reduce their chances of having a fatal coronary by one-quarter (like those healthy Glaswegians in the WOSCOPS study) or by 41 per cent (like those Swedes). But what does this actually mean for the individual? Here we encounter that 'elegant mischief' already considered in the cholestyramine trial, the alchemy by which molehills are transformed into mountains. Tables 4.2 and 4.3 reveal all. Starting with Table 4.2, this gives us along the top line the impressive relative risk reduction for cardiac deaths, and below the considerably more modest 'absolute' benefits.

Table 4.2 The striking difference between the 'relative' and 'absolute' benefit of statins in reducing the risk of cardiac deaths in the WOSCOPS and 4S trials

	WOSCOPS Cardiac deaths	4S Cardiac deaths
Relative rate reduction	−27%	−41%
Absolute rate reduction	−0.42%	−3.5%

To learn how these figures were derived we turn to Table 4.3, starting with the 'primary' prevention WOSCOPS trial.

We note at the top that the numbers in the trial are almost equally divided between those on placebo (3293) and on a statin (3302). There were fifty-two cardiac deaths in the former group, giving a rate of 1.6 per cent; subtract the thirty-eight in those

Table 4.3 The results of the WOSCOPS and the 4S trials

WOSCOPS	Placebo (n=3293)	Rate %	Statin (n=3302)	Rate %
Cardiac deaths	52	1.6	38	1.2

4S TRIAL	Placebo (n=2223)	Rate %	Statin (n=2221)	Rate %
Cardiac deaths	189	8.5	111	5.0

taking a statin, a rate of 1.2 per cent, and this works out at four-teen fewer in numbers and a lower rate of 0.4 per cent. And that 0.4 per cent is indeed a quarter of the 1.6 per cent in the placebo group – hence 'statins reduce the risk of a fatal coronary by a quarter'. But for the individual, the absolute benefit is indeed 0.4 per cent, i.e. less than half a person for every one hundred treated, one person for every two hundred and fifty. Thus, while it is indeed correct, as the press release announcing the results of the trial claimed, that 'For those with a high cholesterol pravas-tatin rapidly reduces the risk of having a fatal coronary by 27 per cent', it would have been no less true to point out that 250 men must swallow 357,000 tablets for five years to save one of them from a fatal coronary, or (which is the same thing) to increase their chances of not having a fatal coronary from 98.4 per cent to 98.8 per cent. By contrast, the same calculations for 'secondary' prevention in the 4S Trial give a 3.5 per cent reduction in abso-lute risk of a fatal coronary (8.5 minus 5), which though vastly less impressive than the 40 per cent relative figure, some might still consider worthwhile. They might perhaps be slightly more dubious if their doctor, before prescribing statins, put it to them in a rather different way: 'If a hundred people like you do not take statins for five years, ninety-two will live and eight will die. Whether you will be one of the ninety-two or one of the eight, I cannot tell. If a hundred people like you take a statin every day for five years, ninety-five will live and five will die. Again, I can't tell whether you will be one of the ninety-five or one of the five.'

There are, needless to say, numerous ways in which drug companies can spin the results of their trials so as to produce the desired finding. But one further instance, though an important one, must suffice. Those aged seventy and over should be a prime target for 'growing' the statin market, as cholesterol levels tend to rise modestly with age – which for a substantial proportion mean that they are above the threshold set by the guidelines for initiating treatment. This group, however, had been excluded from the early statin trials so there was no direct evidence as to the drugs' efficacy or whether indeed the benefits might be offset by the greater likelihood of their experiencing side effects. Hence the catchily titled PROSPER trial (PROspective Study of pravastatin), launched in the late nineties by Professor James Shepherd of Glasgow Royal Infirmary – who had also organised the very influential WOSCOPS trial – and involving 5000 men and women between the ages of seventy and eighty-two with a history of (or risk factors for) heart disease. After three years, those taking pravastatin had been rewarded with 'relatively' one fifth (21 per cent) fewer fatal coronaries (see Table 4.4). This result, Professor Shepherd argued, 'extended to elderly individuals the benefits of statins already demonstrated for the middle aged'. All very satisfactory.

Table 4.4 The results of the PROSPER trial

	Placebo (n=2913)	Rate %	Pravastatin (n=2891)	Rate %	Relative risk reduction	Absolute risk reduction
Cardiac deaths	122	4.2	94	3.3	−21%	−0.9%
Total mortality	306	10.5	298	10.2	−2.8%	−0.3%

But the results expressed in absolute terms, at 0.9 per cent, were predictably much more modest. There are two further significant omissions in the summary of the results that would be of interest to 'the elderly' and indeed their doctors. First, that modest 0.9 per cent benefit *only* applied to men, as the women in the study taking pravastatin had the same number of fatal coronaries as those taking the placebo. And second *there was almost no overall difference in survival* (306 deaths overall for placebo; 298 for statins), the fewer coronary fatalities in those taking pravastatin being offset by an increase in those who succumbed to cancer instead. The probable explanation is as follows. Both heart disease and cancer are strongly influenced by age, being much commoner in the 'elderly'. Hence, the very modest benefit of statins in protecting against heart disease in the elderly allows them to die from some other cause – such as cancer.

Thus, rather than PROSPER 'extending the benefits' of statins to the elderly, it would be just as accurate to say that pravastatin reduces the risk of having a fatal heart attack in men by 0.9 per cent, but not in women, and does not prolong life. Put this way, there cannot be many (or indeed any) of the 'elderly' who would willingly agree to take a statin indefinitely – but millions do, without, of course, having had the opportunity to give their 'informed consent'.

This ingenious spinning of the benefits of statins is considerably less than half the story. For while the vast majority of the millions now taking statins gain no benefit from doing so, they are *all* at the same time vulnerable to the iatrogenic illnesses that statins might cause. These are familiar enough, whether from reading of those 'miraculous' recoveries from decrepitude described by Roger Andrews following his statin-free excursion to Hawaii, or from personal experience, or that of friends and relatives. It would be a miracle if interfering with the synthesis of a biological compound as important as cholesterol did *not* have adverse effects in a substantial proportion of those taking statins. It is thus more than perplexing when we scrutinise the reports of those clinical trials to discover they are apparently very rare, with just 1 per cent experiencing 'adverse effects'. They might at least be expected to be rather more frequent among older persons, but a further oddity of the PROSPER study is that those taking statins were no more likely to experience adverse effects than those on the placebo – with almost equal numbers experiencing, for example, muscular aches and pains. This, it is scarcely necessary to point out, is staggeringly improbable.

Nonetheless, the common perception among doctors, understandably in view of the above, is that statins are 'remarkably safe' and well-tolerated. This in turn has been a major factor in their willingness to prescribe them so freely. That presumption of safety would also, as can be imagined, mean they overlook the possibility that statins might be the culprit for their patients' puzzling symptoms – well illustrated by the experience of Dr Andrew Bamji, Consultant Rheumatologist at Queen Mary's

Hospital Sidcup, who only came to appreciate the scale of the problem when he experienced those adverse effects himself.

'As a rheumatologist, my job is to help people with joint problems and arthritic complaints. So, it was with some irony that I diagnosed myself with tenosynovitis – a severe tendon inflammation I often treat in my patients. This occurred at the front of my shin – a highly unusual place – so I decided to do some research into what might have triggered this. I was amazed to discover the only other related case was linked to a patient on statins – which I had been taking for a couple of months following a high cholesterol reading. Intrigued by the connection, I decided to stop them to see what happened. Within a couple of weeks, the pain had gone. I returned to my GP and over successive months tried various other statins but each form of the drug caused terrible problems including night cramp, muscle pain, severe muscle disorders known as myopathy and general fatigue. In fact, I became so tired I couldn't lift anything when I was gardening or even walk the half mile from my home to the centre of town.'

And then the crunch: 'I began to realise that many of my patients with problems such as polymyalgia, pain, stiffness and tenderness in the muscles, were on statins. When I advised them to stop taking their medication their problems went away.'

Following this article, in which Dr Bamji described his profound insight into the iatrogenic cause of so many of his patients' distressing symptoms, 'I had a deluge of letters describing similar experiences. All railed against the difficulty of getting their doctor to listen and understand that there really was a problem.'

My views on this matter are coloured by all those letters and emails mentioned in the opening chapter, a few extracts from which convey some sense of the gravity of doctors' failure to recognise this pervasive, but readily reversible reason for their patients' medical problems.

The insistence that patients continue to take their medicines despite their clearly adverse effects is baffling as with this seventy-year-old man with Type 2 diabetes in whom statins induced a marked change in personality:

'My doctor prescribed statins after a blood test for cholesterol. I was told the government had ruled that statins be prescribed to all those like myself with Type 2 diabetes over a certain level. The effect they had on me was a complete change of personality. I had been happily married for 41 years but became a complete monster. I knew I was being horrible to my dear wife but was unable to control my verbal attacks on her and the poor woman was reduced to tears; it was awful. It was only after speaking to a neighbour whose husband had also been prescribed statins who told me about his unusually snappy behaviour I realised they could be the cause. I stopped taking them and am pleased to say within a week I was a different man and we remain very happily married. When I told my doctor I would no longer take statins she said I must continue, it was a government ruling – nevertheless I ignored her. My friend not only suffered personality problems but also muscle wastage. After giving up the statins he returned to his usual fit golfing self.'

The misattribution of statin iatrogenesis to 'old age' is a recurring theme:

'In May this year my GP doubled my dose of atorvastatin and there were three side effects which immediately became apparent – a sharp deterioration in my short-term memory, frequent muscle ache, particularly around the torso, and the loss of libido. He tends to think these are a product of old age, but the onset soon after the doubling of the dose is too much of a coincidence for me.'

And so too is outright denial:

'I have been on 40mg of simvastatin since I had a heart attack about four years ago. I suffer from muscle pains and short-term memory problems. I saw my doctor recently and asked him directly whether there were any side effects of statins. He said, without qualification, no. I checked with the leaflet on my next prescription that lists quite a collection of possible side effects but says they may only occur in one in a thousand patients. How, I wonder, do they come to this figure?'

The medical enthusiasm for statins despite doctors' recognising that they are responsible for their patients' symptoms is really quite extraordinary:

'My husband went from a very fit man of 74 to a near invalid within the space of six months after being diagnosed with angina. He quickly recovered after an angioplasty and the fitting of two stents. Statins were prescribed and within a short period he was unable to walk around the lake we live near, had appalling muscle cramps in his legs and generally felt very ill. He contacted his specialist who told him to stop the statins for a few weeks and then resume on a half dose.

He was fine until he recommended the statins whereupon the whole thing started again. From that time, about a year ago, he has refused to take the statins despite his GP and specialist urging him to do so and has been totally fit – holidaying abroad and the UK, walking, gardening, etc.'

It may be necessary for relatives to take unilateral action:

'My husband was prescribed statins some years ago. I have watched him suffer from increasing pain, fatigue and depression to the point that he wondered if it was worth waking up in the morning. Having read reports in the newspapers I, together with a friend, persuaded him to stop taking them for a while as an experiment. Within a few weeks he is walking anything up to five miles a day, the pain is diminished and he is quite fun to live with again! Can this be just coincidence?'

Finally, the cautionary accounts of a pharmacist and a general practitioner who both had to discover statins' adverse effects for themselves:

'I am a male retired pharmacist aged seventy-three. In 1997 I had a heart attack and a stent fitted in Southampton General Hospital. On discharge from hospital I was put on the usual cocktail of drugs including atorvastatin. I experienced a gradual build-up of aches and pains and my long-term memory also deteriorated which I attributed to age. When I read your article on statins I began to wonder if these and a lot of other symptoms – constipation, indigestion, insomnia, dizziness, joint pain, weight gain, tiredness – could be due to a decade's worth of atorvastatin. A review of my medication was due and I suggested to the nurse that I discontinue it for three months to which she agreed. Within 48 hours all my aches and pains had gone. I am now approximately a month into the trial and cannot remember when I felt so well.'

And the GP:

'In May 2006 I suffered a heart attack and was started on the usual cocktail of drugs including simvastatin. I took my aches and pains and the general feeling I can only describe of being twenty years older mentally and physically as par for the course after a heart attack. I returned to work after three months. My partner began to notice errors creeping into my work such as not dealing with blood test results correctly and poor concentration. I eventually consulted my own GP and stopped the statin. Within seven days my concentration and energy levels had returned to normal. Like most GPs I had been following guide-lines and increasing patients' doses of simvastatin to 40mg where needed. My own experience has radically altered my views on this form of mass medication. The blinkered specialists' view that lowering cholesterol has to be good for you is false. This medication has effects not fully disclosed nor yet investigated.'

These poignant accounts speak for themselves, and would more than suggest their reported 'rarity' in these clinical trials is quite as misleading as the exaggeration of their benefits. Of this, more anon. For the moment one may note that those who have sought to assess the issue independently – outside the context of drug company-sponsored trials – have come to a rather different conclusion. Thus, a survey of almost 8000 French statin users found that muscle-related symptoms were ten times higher than those recorded in the clinical trials. Researchers scrutinising the medical records of half a million Danish citizens for reports of severe pain in the limbs from disturbed functioning of the sensory nerves (peripheral neuropathy) found it to be fourteen times commoner in those using statins. A search of the US Food and Drug Administration's database for adverse effects associated with just one brand, atorvastatin, identified 2000 cases of 'serious cognitive dysfunction', 222 reports of 'dementia', 523 of disorientation and 602 of 'a confusional state'. This was more than mere 'association', for as Professor Beatrice Colomb found in a detailed study of patients self-reporting statin-related memory and cognitive problems, 90 per cent were 'markedly improved' within a couple of weeks of stopping their medication – including several misdiagnosed as having dementia. They included

'A retired academic who had developed rapidly progressive severe cognitive loss. He could no longer read a page of text, recall what he had just said, or recognise associates he had known closely for decades and was diagnosed with rapidly progressive Alzheimer's disease. His family discontinued his simvastatin and on his next evaluation – for participation in an Alzheimer's drug trial – he was informed he no longer met criteria for Alzheimer's, nor indeed dementia. Subjective "full" recovery took approximately two years by when he had resumed his daily reading of three national newspapers.'

The general impression from all this would be that a substantial proportion, perhaps one in ten or more, experience in some form severe adverse effects, considerably more than the 1 per cent reported in those drug company-sponsored trials – further testimony to the way, as alleged, they present the results of their trials not just to accentuate the positive but also to play down the negative.

Still, such devious methods could scarcely on their own explain why so many of those who currently take statins have been misled into supposing their benefits to be so much greater, the harms so much less, than they really are. They are, after all, persuaded (or cajoled or coerced) to do so by doctors within whose ranks, and the most ardent advocates of 'statins for all', are the by now familiar and influential epidemiologists. In 2012 the most prominent advocate of all, Professor Rory Collins of Oxford University, raised the ante still further, asserting that statins should now be routinely given to everyone over the age of fifty, widening the net by a further five million over and above the seven million adults in Britain already taking them. This assertion of the seemingly inestimable good of lowering cholesterol (albeit by pharmacological means) brings us to the closing episode of the statin saga – the third of the trio of closely related and perplexing epidemiological contributions (after the 'population theory' and the diet-heart thesis) to the pharmaceutical industry's goal of mass medicalisation.

This is how it came about. Soon after the publication of that first trial back in 1994 involving more than 4,000 Swedes (the 4S Trial) that (ostensibly) reduced the risk of a fatal coronary by 40 per cent, Professor Collins, together with Richard Peto, also of Oxford University, anticipated the drug companies might provide generous financial support to an independent academic institution which could synthesise the results of the many similar trials planned for the future. And indeed they did, perhaps hoping to allay the not unreasonable suspicion of bias in their own interpretation of the findings. Accordingly, they agreed to provide the Cholesterol Treatment Trialists' Collaboration (CTTC), as it is known, with exclusive access to the voluminous original (or raw) data generated by the trials.

This is a costly business for, as can be imagined, checking the outcomes in tens of thousands of participants in those clinical trials is a formidable task. How costly is not known, as drug company financial support for the CTTC has never been declared – though its parent organisation, the Oxford University Clinical Trial Services Unit, has received £268 million over the past twenty years, £218 million contributed by just one company, Merck.

Still, it would be money well spent, as the CTTC's olympian overview of what eventually turned out to be twenty-seven statin trials involving more than 170,000 participants should, it was expected, iron out any inconsistencies and irregularities to produce a definitive answer as to just how effective statins were, and in whom.

Professor Collins's independent interpretation proved very favourable indeed. Statins, it transpired, in a review published in 2012, are *so* effective, they reduce the 'relative risk' of not just heart attacks but strokes as well, in both men and women, young and old, in those with normal and raised cholesterol levels. They work, it appears, equally well for primary and secondary prevention in those at 'high' and those at 'low' risk of cardiovascular disease. Fulfilling Henry Gadsden's dream, they work, in short, for everyone. This verdict, noted one of Professor Collins's collaborators, 'settles once and for all previous uncertainties about whether healthy, middle-aged people should benefit from taking statins – that greatly exceed any known harms'. Soon after publication of these rather astonishing findings, Professor Collins elaborated further, in a lecture named, appropriately enough, in honour of Geoffrey Rose, the founding father of the 'population approach'. The main impediment to realising the immensely beneficial therapeutic potential of statins for so many, he argued, was an exaggerated fear of their potential harm. 'The reality is that these drugs are safe,' he is quoted as saying, the only proven side effect being a very low risk of muscle damage that is easily outweighed by their benefits. Accordingly, he proposed the criteria for initiating treatment be extended to all who had a greater than one in ten chance of a coronary over the next ten years (a 'coronary risk' of greater than 10 per cent) which would, as noted above, increase the numbers eligible by a further five million.

This notion of 'coronary risk' merits a brief diversion. The initial impetus for the decades-long cholesterol-lowering campaign derived from the certainty that those with markedly raised cholesterol are at increased risk of a coronary. But, as will be recalled, most of those who suffer a heart attack or fatal coronary have normal or near normal cholesterol levels, hence the supposition that their normal levels were in fact 'abnormal' ('the population is sick'), in turn justifying the trend of lowering the threshold for initiating treatment to include a third of all adults. But, the argument went, many more still would benefit if the criteria for prescribing them took into account all the other 'risk factors' for heart disease – smoking (of course), blood pressure, family history and especially age.

It is difficult to take all these other factors into account, so statisticians have devised several methods (or mathematical algorithms) that integrate all these risk factors into a single figure or 'coronary risk score'. The most widely used, the QRisk2 score, could scarcely be easier. The doctor types the patient's details – age, sex, smoking, cholesterol level, etc. – into the computer and up pops a number which then determines whether or not statins should be prescribed.

But the statistical method by which this score is derived is so bafflingly complex one might reasonably wonder as to just how accurately it does predict the likelihood of having a coronary. I quote here a couple of illustrative extracts to emphasise how doctors, when routinely prescribing statins on the basis of their patients' 'score', can have no intellectual understanding of why they are doing so. Thus, starting with the risk factor data from two million patients, Professor of Clinical Epidemiology Julia Hippisley-Cox describes how:

'The observed risk [of heart disease] at ten years was obtained by using the ten-year Kaplan-Meier estimate. We calculated the Brier score (a measure of goodness of fit where lower values indicate better accuracy) using the censoring adjusted version adapted for survival data, D statistic (a measure of discrimination where higher values indicate better discrimination), and an R2 statistic. This is a measure of explained variation where higher values indicate more explained variation. We also calculated the area under the receiver operator curve (ROC) where higher values indicate better discrimination.'

Now these statistical correlations may accurately predict the likelihood of a future coronary, or they may not – for it transpires that 80 per cent of the relevant data for those two million patients was 'incomplete', warranting a further set of statistical adjustments known as 'multiple imputation':

'Our main analyses used multiple imputation to replace miss-ing values for systolic blood pressure, cholesterol, smoking, status and body mass index. Our final model was fitted based on multiply imputed data sets using Rubin's rules to combine effect estimates and estimate standard errors to allow for the uncertainty caused by the missing data, etc., etc.'

Now back to Professor Collins. Prior to the publication of the CTTC analysis in the *Lancet* in 2012, doctors were advised they should prescribe statins to those with a QRisk2 score of 20 per cent or greater – i.e. a one in five chance of having a coronary over the next ten years. That might sound quite serious but means rather that, according to these impenetrable statistical calculations (if they are valid – and how can one tell?), one has an 'estimated' risk, not that one will have a coronary. Anyhow, Professor Collins was so impressed by the findings of his anal-ysis – that statins are not only immensely safe but apparently work for everyone – he proposed the bar for their prescription should be lowered still further, from a one in five risk (20 per cent) to one in ten (10 per cent). Now, as with all illnesses, the older you are the greater the chances of a coronary, so most people in their sixties and over have a QRisk2 score of 10 per cent or more – thus becoming automatically eligible for statins.

It helps to appreciate the implications of this for everyday medicine to imagine a busy GP in his surgery contemplating whether to prescribe a statin to his otherwise healthy patient, Mr Jones in his early seventies. He types in Mr Jones's age, blood pressure, cholesterol level, etc., and up pops a score of, say, 12 per cent, whose statistical derivation neither he nor any other GP in the country could conceivably comprehend. The decision that statins will be of benefit to Mr Jones is of course predicated on Professor Collins's grand synthesis of those twenty-seven trials, whose calculations are not open to public scrutiny and the validity of whose conclusions the GP would be incapable of evaluating. Indeed, the only firm piece of evidence on which he could base his decision is that PROSPER trial in the elderly, where for someone of Mr Jones's age statins reduce the absolute risk of a fatal coronary by 0.9 per cent without reducing overall mortality – i.e. he will not live any longer for taking them. The GP is thus in no position to seek Mr Jones's informed consent, as he himself does not possess the relevant information. He signs a prescription, and urges Mr Jones to take them on the grounds that they have been shown (by clever epidemiologists in Oxford) to be very effective and very safe.

But just how effective and safe are they? They are not what they are cracked up to be, according to Dr John Abramson of Harvard Medical School. '[Professor Collins's] figures might sound good,' he observed in a highly critical review in the *British Medical Journal*, but 'close examination raises questions about both benefits and harm.' They certainly do not improve survival in those taking them for 'primary prevention', and as for strokes and heart disease, 167 people need to take them for five years to prevent one or other of these misfortunes in just one of their number, leaving the remaining 166 exposed to the possible harms for no benefit. Doctors, Dr Abramson suggested, 'would provide a far greater service to their patients by explaining the [modest] magnitude of the benefits and uncertainty about the harms'. And thus, Dr Abramson maintains, the two-thirds of those taking statins who are at 'low risk' of coronary heart disease do not prolong their life by doing so.

The acrimonious arguments, with their claims and counter-claims, rumble on. Contrary to the claim that the CTTC analysis had 'settled [the matter] once and for all', the editor of the *British Medical Journal*, Fiona Godlee, would observe four years later:

> 'Questions about statins continue to emerge from many quarters. How strong is the evidence? How large is the benefit for individuals at lowest risk of heart disease? How well do the trials record common minor side effects? How representative were the trials of women and the elderly? Why is there a discrepancy between the real-life experience of muscle pains and what is reported in the trials? Why have the data for harms not yet been given the same level of scrutiny as the data for benefits?'

Meanwhile – off-piste, as it were, but more than relevant to those 'questions emerging from many quarters' – three significant developments would further undermine the façade of knowledge sustaining 'statins for all'. First, the diet-heart thesis, with its powerful imagery implicating high-fat meat and dairy products in the epidemic of heart disease, became yet more insecure when nutritional researchers from Cambridge University, following an exhaustive review of the evidence, concluded that 'Saturated fats are not associated with coronary heart disease, diabetes or deaths from any cause.' Next, it transpired that the 'coronary risk score' that legitimises the prescription of statins to virtually all over the age of sixty-five overestimates the subsequent risk of a coronary by approximately five-fold. Finally, the striking pattern of the 'rise and fall' of heart disease over the past seventy years has continued its downward trajectory to which the dizzying upward spiral of the twelve-fold increase in prescriptions for statins over the past twenty years has made no discernible contribution (Figure 4.3).

Figure 4.3 The mass prescription of statins has had no discernible impact on the continuing decline in deaths from heart disease in Britain

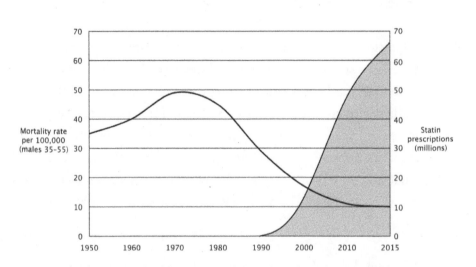

For those who might reasonably wish to extricate themselves from the well-spun web of half-truths that have trapped so many an American physician, Dr David Newman of New York's Mount Sinai Hospital has devised a simple and readily comprehensible pie chart for making an 'informed choice': how many people need to take a statin for one person to benefit? – otherwise known as the Numbers Needed to Treat (NNT) (see Figure 4.4). We have here two pie charts for 'primary' and 'secondary' prevention, with at the centre, prominently displayed for good reason, the very important 'no benefit' figure of 98 per cent and 96 per cent respectively. Then, atop the chart, there is a line giving 'benefits', where we note that for 'primary prevention' statins do not save lives. They will, however, prevent a heart attack in 1 in 104 (0.9 per cent) and a stroke in 1 in 154 (0.4 per cent). Moving to the second pie chart, the figures for those prescribed statins as

'secondary' prevention are considerably better. Here they prolong
life in 1 in 83 (1.2 per cent), and prevent a heart attack in 1 in 39
(2.6 per cent) and a stroke in 1 in 125 (0.8 per cent).

Figure 4.4 Numbers Needed to Treat (NNT)

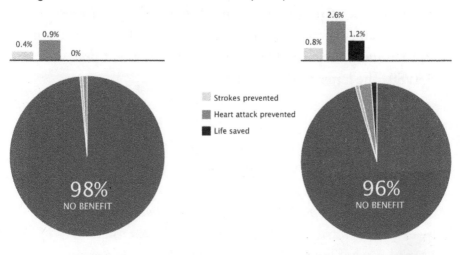

The great merits of Dr Newman's pie charts is that they allow
the individual to make an informed decision depending on his or
her personal inclination. The cautious may well be prepared to take
a statin indefinitely in the hope that they might, for example, be
the one among 104 (primary) or 39 (secondary) for whom statins
prevent a heart attack. But it might be equally reasonable to trust
to fortune and decline to take a statin on the grounds that you will
much more likely be one of the 103 (primary) or 38 (secondary)
who do not benefit. So that's sorted – the take-home message
being that cholesterol, as suggested in the previous chapter, is not
entirely innocent. It does have 'something' to do with heart disease
but, other than for those in whom it is markedly elevated or who
have a history of heart disease, it is not a determinant factor. Were

it to be so, then the benefits of taking statins would be much more generous than the very narrow slivers of those pie charts.

Epilogue

In December 2015, a 79-year-old Bradford woman received the following letter from her family doctor enclosing a prescription for atorvastatin. She had no history of heart disease in her family, a cholesterol level of just 4.9 and blood pressure of 150/80. The letter read as follows:

Dear Caroline

After reviewing your medical record, you have been identified as having a significant risk of developing heart disease in the next ten years. To help reduce your risk, we advise that you now take a statin regularly that can help reduce the risk of stroke and heart attack by a third if taken regularly. They are one of the most researched medicines and there is very strong evidence that they help prevent the conditions described above. They work best if taken long term.

We want to make starting a statin as convenient as possible and to maximise the benefits to your health. Therefore, a statin called atorvastatin has been added to your repeat prescribing list and a prescription will be enclosed with this letter.

Yours sincerely . . .

It is scarcely necessary to point out that every assertion in this letter is either false or misleading, while the possibility that the 'attached prescription' for atorvastatin might cause adverse effects is not mentioned. So much for informed consent. Thus has Henry Gadsden's vision of 'selling to everyone' profoundly compromised medicine's ethical values.

Chapter 5

Diabetes: A Catalogue of Errors

'I had a fasting blood sugar test as part of a well-man check. The result was "high" and my GP unhesitatingly diagnosed Type 2 diabetes. This was despite my protesting I felt as fit as a fiddle. The dreaded scenario explained to me was that there were probably millions of people walking around with undiagnosed diabetes, showing no symptoms at all, feeling just like me, fit and healthy. But the condition was there, quietly destroying their eyesight, nerves and feet and much else. One day their systems will not be able to take any more and the serious symptoms of diabetes will become apparent. They too will then need to be put on medication but irreversible damage will have been done. However, because I had been diagnosed early, medication could prevent all this happening and I could live a healthy, happy life. Lucky old me!'

Diabetes is the third of the pharmaceutical industry's trio of golden geese – large numbers, lifelong treatment and a bonanza of blood sugar-lowering drugs. Still, diabetes is qualitatively different from having hypertension or 'raised' cholesterol that can be remedied by the simple expedient of taking one or several pills per day. Rather, it is an ancient, life-changing illness requiring adherence to a dietary regime that may not be congenial, a painful thumb-pricking ritual, and a life lived under constant medical scrutiny to detect the early signs of those grievous complications.

It is quite different in another way, for while we will encounter the now familiar themes of over-diagnosis and over-medication, the current 'epidemic' of diabetes has the distinction of being the single most comprehensive iatrogenic catastrophe of all. Really? Here the issue of credibility, as mentioned in the Introduction, is particularly acute. The account of the rise of polypharmacy and its consequences is so contrary to the common perception of medicine as a beneficent science-based discipline that any reasonable person might suppose, 'That can't possibly be true.' And no more so than here. How could legions of knowledgeable, experienced specialists, nutritional scientists, dieticians and general practitioners conceivably be guilty of fostering 'an iatrogenic catastrophe'? Still, as some may be aware, the last few years have witnessed an extraordinary situation where many of those with diabetes have defied the authoritative advice of their medical advisers, and in doing so have transformed their lives immeasurably for the better. Their experience is the most persuasive instance of the imperative for 'ordinary people' to make their own independent judgement on the medical advice they receive.

The cause of diabetes, as all know, relates to the action of the hormone insulin, secreted by a small cluster of cells (the Islets of Langerhans) in the pancreas, to control the uptake of the body's 'fuel', glucose, into its cells. When the amount of insulin is either deficient or insufficient for the body's needs, the level of glucose ('blood sugar') rises but cannot be utilised. The body's cells are thus starved of glucose despite its abundance in the bloodstream. Hence the description of diabetes as 'starvation in the midst of plenty'. Furthermore, its high concentration in the blood sucks water out of the tissues that (by the action of osmosis) become dehydrated, the water being excreted in large volumes in the urine. Hence the three cardinal symptoms of diabetes: weight loss (starvation in the midst of plenty), thirst and excessive urination – vividly described by the Greek physician Aretaeus of Cappadocia in the second century AD: 'Life is disgusting and thirst unquenchable. If for a time they abstain from drinking the mouth becomes parched and the body dry; the viscera seems as if scorched up ... the melting is rapid, the death speedy.'

Almost two thousand years later, the treatment of this terrible illness would be the first, and arguably most dramatic, of the many triumphs of modern medicine.

In 1921, thirteen-year-old Leonard Thompson was admitted to Ward H of Toronto General Hospital, subsequently described by one of his doctors as 'a pathetic, emaciated figure lying quietly in his bed, too weak to show any interest in the activities of a large busy ward. All of us knew he was doomed.' But he was not. Two scientists, Frederick Banting and Charles Best, had recently extracted purified insulin from a dog's pancreas and were looking for a patient to treat. Leonard Thompson was the obvious candidate. 'The results were certain. This dying boy literally came back to life.' It was as a 'sturdy young man' he was discharged from hospital two months later.

Since then, while the cause of the destruction of those Islets of Langerhans responsible for Leonard Thompson's Type 1 diabetes remains obscure, its treatment has become ever more sophisticated with the introduction of a genetically modified form of human insulin and infusion pumps to ensure a constant level of the hormone in the body. No longer 'doomed', the life expectancy of today's Leonard Thompsons approximates to that of their contemporaries.

This chapter is concerned with the second form of diabetes (Type 2 or maturity onset), different in many ways from Type 1 other than in the shared feature of raised blood sugar level. The deficiency of insulin in Type 1 is absolute, hence the need for its replacement. By contrast Type 2 is an 'insufficiency' disease; the Islets of Langerhans are intact, but the amount of insulin they produce is insufficient to meet the demands placed upon it. This is an illness of the middle-aged and elderly (hence 'maturity onset'), most of whom, being overweight, are burdened with an excess of fat cells whose requirement for insulin outstrips its supply. Most are only identified as having the condition following a routine blood test though they may recognise in retrospect those classic symptoms of thirst and excess urination (albeit in much milder form) or the cause of their being troubled by recurrent bouts of boils or abscesses 'fed' by those raised sugar levels. For some, too, the combination of raised levels of both sugar and insulin in the blood induces what is known as the 'metabolic syndrome', a generalised disturbance of the body's biochemistry characterised by fatty infiltration of the liver, raised amounts of the fats cholesterol and triglyceride and raised blood pressure.

The remedy for Type 2 diabetes is (obviously enough) to lose that surplus weight, for then their previous 'insufficiency' of insulin becomes 'sufficient' to ensure the uptake of glucose into the cells. It does not matter how that weight loss is achieved; vegans can do it as readily as meat eaters, as long as they restrict the amount of calories they consume.

Nonetheless, raised levels of blood glucose, the salient feature of diabetes, are inevitably compounded by the consumption of sugars – or the starchy (carbohydrate) foods such as bread, pasta, rice and potatoes that are most readily converted into sugar. Thus, logically, a 'low carbohydrate diet' cutting back on starchy foods is the preferred method of weight loss. And very effective it is too, as famously demonstrated by William Banting, carpenter and coffin maker to the rich and famous, in his elegantly written pamphlet 'Letter on corpulence addressed to the public', published in 1863. Though just 5ft 5in (1.6m) tall, Banting was at 14st 6lb (92 kg) almost four stone (25 kg) overweight and 'brought to a low impoverished state by many obnoxious boils and two formidable carbuncles':

> 'I could not stoop to tie my shoes or attend to the little offices humanity requires without considerable pain and difficulty that only the corpulent can understand. I have been compelled to go down the stairs slowly, backward, to save the jar of increased weight on the knee and ankle joints and have been obliged to puff and blow over every slight exertion, particularly that of going up stairs.'

He had tried every conceivable means to lose weight, including acquiring 'a good heavy safe boat I would row for a couple of hours every morning':

'I have tried sea air, bathing in various localities with much walking exercise; riding on horseback; the waters and climate of Leamington many times, as well as those of Cheltenham and Harrogate and have spared no trouble nor expense in consultations with the best authorities in the land. All in vain.'

In his early sixties, Banting became increasingly hard of hearing, prompting him to consult Dr William Harvey, Fellow of the Royal College of Surgeons and an ear, nose and throat specialist. Dr Harvey had recently returned from Paris where he had attended a series of lectures by the eminent Dr Claude Bernard, whose investigations into the role of the liver in maintaining a constant level of sugar in the blood would lead to his formulation of the grand unifying physiological principle of homeostasis.

Dr Harvey advised Banting, on the basis of Bernard's investigations, that he should change his 'diet', which till then had consisted of:

'Breakfast: bread and milk for breakfast, or a pint of tea with plenty of milk and sugar, and buttered toast.
   Lunch: meat, beer, bread and pastry.
   Tea: a meal similar to breakfast.
   Supper: generally a fruit tart or bread and milk.'

Dr Harvey proposed eliminating starchy foods, particularly sugar, bread, milk, beer and potatoes, allowing his patient 'up to six ounces of bacon, beef, mutton, venison, kidneys, fish or any form of poultry; the fruit of any pudding – but without the pastry; any vegetable except potato; at dinner two or three glasses of good claret, sherry or madeira; tea without milk or sugar'. Champagne, port and beer were forbidden and he could only eat one ounce of toast.

Within nine months Banting had lost three stone. 'I have not felt so well as now for the last twenty years,' he wrote, noting he had 'suffered no inconvenience' from his dietary regime. He could now 'come down the stairs forward naturally with perfect ease and perform every necessary office for myself'. He maintained a normal weight on this dietary regime for the rest of his life, dying at the ripe age of eighty-one.

William Harvey's dietary prescription for his very grateful patient is, in modern parlance, known as a low carbohydrate/ high fat (LCHF) diet. This is slightly confusing as it is not particularly 'high' in fat; rather, when the amount of carbohydrate is restricted then the contribution of saturated fat in the form of meat, milk, butter, cheese and other dairy products is indeed relatively 'high'.

The merit of the LCHF diet for those with Type 2 diabetes is scarcely rocket science, vividly demonstrated, more scientifically than in William Banting's 'Letter', in a study from 1978 conducted by Dr D. R. Hadden of Belfast's Royal Victoria Hospital. The 'subjects' were fifty-seven patients with Type 2 diabetes, each on average 25lb (11 kg) overweight. The results graphically portrayed (Figure 5.1) could scarcely be more compelling: over a period of eight months, they lost on average 20lb (9 kg), paralleled by a decline in their elevated blood sugar levels from a diabetic state (12 mmol/L) back within the normal range (7 mmol/L). 'Carbohydrate restriction is a determining factor in the control of the diabetic state,' Dr Hadden observed.

This brings us to the conundrum posed by the much commented-on diabetes 'epidemic': why, given that it is for many

Figure 5.1 The impressive weight loss of patients with Type 2 diabetes on a low carbohydrate diet is paralleled by a fall in the blood sugar level back into the normal range

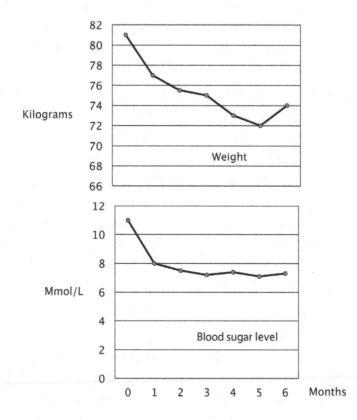

a reversible condition, the numbers so diagnosed should have risen four-fold over the past few decades – up from 800,000 to almost 3 million in Britain and from 5 million in 20 million in the United States – with a similar four-fold increase in spending on diabetic medicines – up from £70 million to £277 million in Britain, and from $3.8 billion to $17.8 billion in the United States.

The dynamic behind this 'epidemic' has much in common with the similar rise in the numbers deemed eligible for treatment with statins and antihypertensives. We start with the now familiar technique (or ploy) of markedly increasing the scope for medical intervention by reducing downwards, in numerical terms, the cut-off point for its diagnosis, which in 1979 was set at 7.7 mmol/L. Then in 1998 it was decreed that the threshold be lowered to 7.0 mmol/L, increasing at a stroke the numbers with the condition in Britain by a further 300,000 and in the United States by 1.6 million.

In 2011 the diagnostic criterion was switched from the blood glucose level to measuring the glucose level in the red blood cells (glycated haemoglobin, or HbA1c), which ostensibly provides a more accurate measurement of the effects of raised blood sugar on the tissues of the body. Family doctors applying this new criterion – an HbA1c of 6.5 per cent or more – found they were diagnosing diabetes in twice as many patients as previously. Thus the 'epidemic' is in one sense an artefact of measurement. The vast majority self-evidently have no symptoms of the illness; indeed, like the gentleman cited at the opening of this chapter, they may well feel 'perfectly fit'. Nonetheless those above the threshold are diagnosed as having diabetes on the grounds that they are at risk of subsequently developing its 'complications' – heart disease, blindness, kidney failure, etc. – which can be prevented or minimised by reducing the blood sugar (by dietary means or medication) to or below the arbitrary definition of 'normal'.

Still, the almost quadrupling of the numbers diagnosed with Type 2 diabetes over the past twenty-five years does reflect a genuine increase in incidence, paralleled as it is by a similar rise in the proportion of the population who are fatter than they should be. Those who are overweight, as noted above, are particularly prone because they produce insufficient insulin for their needs. And, whatever the cause – whether eating too much or the 'wrong type of food', or taking too little exercise – people have on average become a lot heavier over the past three decades. Surveys consistently reveal that 'the prevalence of obesity' has increased from 15 per cent of the adult population in 1980 to 30 per cent in 2015 – or one in three. Thus, the combination of the lowered thresholds and increasing prevalence of obesity would seem to provide a satisfactory explanation for the current 'epidemic'.

This leaves unanswered that very puzzling question as to why, given the reversibility of diabetes with weight loss and the LCHF diet, this should have happened at all. Something must have happened to trigger this remorseless rise over the past three decades. As indeed it has. Astonishingly, and almost impossible to believe in retrospect, the common-sense advice to those with diabetes that they should restrict the amount of starchy foods they consume was reversed. In one of the most remarkable turnabouts in the history of medicine, an influential group of nutritionists and epidemiologists in their report 'Dietary recommendations for diabetics for the 1980s' condemned the low carbohydrate diet as positively harmful, indeed the worst conceivable for those with diabetes. 'Many of the traditional beliefs concerning the diabetic diet are unproven or wrong.' How so?

Here it is necessary to take a deep breath and return to that time back in the early 1980s when, as will be recalled, epidemiologists had convinced themselves – and sought to convince the public – of their grand all-encompassing theory that a 'high fat' diet was the primary cause of most common illnesses such as heart disease and cancer, as dramatically summarised in that article in *The Times* cited earlier: 'Leaders of the medical profession now have come to speak of the rate of premature death in this country in apocalyptic terms – as a holocaust, which medicine can do nothing to check. Food is the main single underlying cause of disease.'

The central difficulty for those 'leaders of the medical profession' in promoting this all-encompassing theory was the failure (as described in some detail in Chapter 3) of the major 'lifestyle intervention' studies intended to demonstrate that cajoling people into reducing their consumption of meat, milk and dairy products would indeed reduce their risk of heart disease. They had accordingly resorted to the standard device of the 'expert report' to assert by fiat what their scientific investigations had so singularly failed to confirm.

The gist of their recommendations is by now familiar enough – everyone should eat less meat, replace butter with margarine, and reduce consumption of eggs and cheese and so on in favour of 'healthy' carbohydrates – which would, by lowering their cholesterol levels, reduce their risk of heart disease. They could and would do no such thing. Humans survive and flourish irrespective of whether they have a 'high fat' diet (as, famously, the Masai) or, like vegetarians, a 'high carbohydrate' diet. So, fiddling around with what is on the dinner plate will make zero difference, for better or for worse, to their general health. The only group in whom it might matter are those with diabetes – and here epidemiologists were compelled by their commitment to the diet-heart thesis to suppose that their undoubtedly increased liability to heart disease must be due to their 'cutting back' on carbohydrates to control their blood sugar levels and making up the difference with 'high fat meat and dairy products'. They thus had no alternative other than to insist, in their 'Dietary recommendations for the 1980s', that 'many of the traditional beliefs are unproven or wrong' and turn conventional wisdom on its head by advising that those with diabetes, along with everyone else, should favour 'healthy' carbohydrates over 'wicked' saturated fats.

This necessarily required them to finesse the common-sense arguments in favour of restricting starchy foods and the unarguable scientific evidence – such as Dr Hadden's study described above – demonstrating its merits. First, they claimed it did not matter how much carbohydrate was consumed so long as the blood sugar level was controlled by medication. Or as they put it, 'When treatment [with drugs] is adequate the body can adapt to any amount of carbohydrate in the diet.' But what about those who had been successfully controlling their diabetes on a low carbohydrate diet? Surely they should continue to do so? Apparently not. Its effectiveness, they maintained, was not due 'to a restriction of carbohydrates *per se*' but rather to a reduction in the total amount of calories of food consumed, which could as readily be achieved by eating less meat and dairy products. There was, they conceded, 'no proof' this dramatic reversal of the previous dietary advice would reduce the risk of heart disease in those with diabetes, but nonetheless they asserted 'These recommendations are based on the evidence available at the present time and will be reviewed as new facts come to light.' They never have been.

Thus, it was decreed that in future those with diabetes should adopt the same 'healthy' diet as recommended for everyone else – in defiance of the self-evident truth that they are *not* the same as everyone else, the defining feature of their illness being 'carbohydrate intolerance'. And so it has been ever since that those with diabetes, encouraged to 'include starchy carbohydrate foods (bread, pasta, potatoes, noodles, rice and cereals) at each meal', have struggled to lose weight and lower their levels of blood sugar, relying instead, as those experts recommended more than thirty years ago, on drugs to do so. This, as much as anything else, accounts for the four-fold increase in Type 2 diabetes over the past twenty-five years – an iatrogenic catastrophe of epic proportions.

As will be seen, wiser counsels have belatedly begun to prevail. But we turn now to two further misfortunes to befall those with Type 2 diabetes. The burgeoning epidemic and dire effects of that now officially endorsed high carbohydrate diet created an ever-expanding market for the pharmaceutical industry to promote its drugs under the slogan 'tighter control'. The argument, put simply, runs as follows. While most of those with Type 2 diabetes are 'fit and well', though needing medication to control their elevated blood sugar levels, it is an insidious illness that, over time, damages the lining of the arteries, reducing the blood flow to vital organs and resulting in the complications mentioned above. These fall into two categories. The first are the macrovascular, affecting the large (macro) arteries to the heart, limbs and brain, predisposing the sufferer to heart disease, pain in the legs on exertion (claudication) and stroke. The second are the microvascular, affecting the small (micro) blood vessels, including those in the retina at the back of the eye, the nerves and kidney – resulting in impaired vision, neuropathy and kidney damage. Thus, the sooner diabetes is diagnosed the better, by measuring everyone's HbA1c levels in anticipation of finding all those with 'hidden' diabetes that warrant appropriate treatment.

But that is not all, for it is reasonable to assume the more effective the treatment in lowering blood sugar levels (the 'tighter the control'), the greater the likelihood of minimising or indeed preventing damage to those large and small arteries and the complications associated with them. The symptoms of diabetes begin to become apparent above an HbA1c of 9 per cent; while it may be relatively straightforward (and indeed necessary) to reduce that to 8 per cent, would it not be better to lower it to 7.5 per cent or 7 per cent, all the way down to the current 'normal' threshold of 6.5 per cent?

This pursuit of ever tighter control does however have its drawbacks as it requires treating ever more people with ever more drugs and keeping them under ever closer scrutiny to ensure the desired HbA1c target is being achieved. This can mean that rather than 'living with' diabetes, it comes to dominate the patient's life. And the more drugs taken, the greater the likelihood of excess lowering of the blood sugar to cause a 'hypo', reversible with a sweetened drink or glucose infusion but which may have more serious consequences – as American physician Dr Gilbert Welch describes in his appropriately titled book, *Overdiagnosed: Making People Sick in the Pursuit of Health*:

'This is not a happy story. Mr Roberts was a 74-year-old man whose only major medical problem was severe ulcerative colitis for which he had part of his colon surgically removed. Then, in a routine test, Mr Roberts was found to have an elevated blood sugar level. It wasn't that high, but the finding prompted more testing leading to him being diagnosed with diabetes so, although he had no symptoms, his family doctor started him on glyburide – a drug that lowers blood sugar. The medication worked well.

Six months later he blacked out while driving on the local interstate. His car went off the road and rolled over, shattering his sixth and seventh cervical vertebrae – in other words he broke his neck. The paramedics on the scene measured his blood sugar. It was very low. The medication had worked too well. I'd hate to have been the doctor who prescribed him glyburide.

But I was that doctor. I am not sure what happened. I had used the standard starting dose of medication. He had tolerated it well for almost half a year. Maybe he hadn't eaten normally that day; maybe he had the flu or some stomach virus. I don't know. Mr Roberts was in the hospital for over a month. I felt terrible and – it goes without saying – I didn't restart the glyburide. Mr Roberts is now ninety and is still a patient of mine. He has not been treated for diabetes since the accident, nor has he any complications from diabetes. I think he was over-diagnosed. But he was lucky. There was no permanent injury. He has recovered fully from the problems caused by his unneeded treatment. But I am not sure I have.'

The two leading advocates of 'tightening control' were, predictably, the epidemiologists and the drug companies. The epidemiologists invoked the 'population approach' to argue that the 'target' for HbA1c should be reduced from 7.5 per cent to 7 per cent on the grounds that this would shift the 'average' blood sugar level in the population downwards: so many more would benefit. Put simply, 'the lower the HbA1c the better'. Meanwhile the pharmaceutical industry had not profited as much as they would have wished from the diabetes epidemic as the standard anti-diabetic drugs (such as metformin) had been around for a long time and were no longer patented. The drug companies had, however, invested heavily in developing new (and very costly) drugs that, variously, boosted the amount of insulin secreted by the pancreas or 'sensitised' the tissues to its effects. 'Diabetes is common and current drugs are only partially effective in controlling glucose levels and preventing late complications,' a pharmaceutical industry analyst observed. 'It is therefore expected to remain one of the most attractive growth areas in the global pharmaceutical market – especially with those increasingly demanding guidelines for tighter control.' The 'increasingly demanding' guidelines required initiating treatment with the already mentioned metformin and then moving on through two further stages of intensification with these novel anti-diabetic drugs.

The rationale for 'tighter control' seemed plausible enough, but the crucial question of whether it did indeed help prevent those complications remained unanswered. Theoretically it should, but the publication of three major clinical trials in quick succession, involving over 20,000 patients, comparing 'intensified' with standard therapy came to the contrary conclusion. Or, as Professor John Yudkin of London's University College observed, there is 'no increase in life expectancy and quality of life from intensified diabetic therapy.' There was, to be sure, a small protective effect against kidney damage in one of the trials and a 1.4 per cent fall in (non-fatal) heart attacks, but 'Tighter control conferred no benefit in reducing the incidence of coronary mortality, strokes or total deaths.' The pursuit of 'tighter control' resulted predictably in a much higher incidence of 'hypos' and, alarmingly, in one trial a higher mortality rate (257 versus 203 'deaths from all causes'). Put another way, the pursuit of tighter control in a thousand patients treated for five years might be expected to prevent eight non-fatal heart attacks, but would cause an additional forty-seven hypoglycaemic episodes of sufficient severity as to warrant medical intervention. 'When the risk of complications is low,' observed Professor Yudkin, 'and the burden of treatment correspondingly high, it will do more harm than good.'

The further misfortune to befall those with diabetes concerned the 'metabolic syndrome', that combination of disorders of the metabolism in the overweight that, besides raising the blood sugar level, is also associated with increased levels of fats (cholesterol and triglyceride) in the blood, and with hypertension. This, as can be imagined, added yet further to the burden of medication, requiring, besides one, two or three anti-diabetic drugs, both a cholesterol-lowering statin and one or more blood pressure-lowering drugs.

For all that, many of those with Type 2 diabetes would not require any medication at all were they on a low carbohydrate diet – which brings us to the final episode in this tragedy of errors: the patients' revolt. The folly of those 'Dietary recommendations for the 1980s' (so obvious in retrospect) can seem difficult to comprehend – how could they have gone unchallenged for so long? But here the wisdom of hindsight can be deceptive for it underestimates just how deeply the notion of the diet-heart thesis, with its immensely powerful imagery, had become entrenched in the medical psyche. The causative role of saturated fat in heart disease, it was persistently reiterated, had been proven 'beyond reasonable doubt'.

Those with diabetes are at increased risk of heart disease. It would thus be foolhardy in the extreme to further compound that risk by ignoring the dietary advice – universally endorsed, it must be emphasised – in favour of taking carbohydrates at every meal. There has, however, always been a dissident minority prepared to do so, despite the opprobrium of their doctors, and been rewarded as a result. They remained a minority until two scientific papers in 2005 initiated the diabetes counter-revolution. The first, no more than a simpler version of Dr Hadden's long-forgotten study from almost thirty years previously, compared the blood sugar levels in ten overweight patients with Type 2 diabetes first on a standard 'healthy' high carbohydrate diet and then on the LCHF. The disparity between the former (who exhibited markedly raised blood sugar levels) and the latter (who fell within the normal range) needs no elaboration. Soon after, Dr Richard Feinman of the State University of New York, having reviewed the findings of all the physiological investigations into the effects of carbohydrate restriction, confirmed it also 'reverted' the metabolic syndrome and thus the need for that combination of anti-diabetic, cholesterol-lowering and blood pressure-lowering drugs.

Meanwhile, the dissident minority who had disputed the medical advice to take 'carbohydrates at every meal' acquired a collective and forceful voice, through the technological marvel of the internet, a social media forum that would allow people 'to share their own experiences about the real-world nature of diabetes'. And in the real world, as the thousands of those who joined the forum attested, they had struggled for years to control their weight and blood sugar levels until switching to the LCHF diet:

'My husband was diagnosed Type 2 and casually told it was not reversible and he would be on drugs for ever. He went onto the low carb diet, lost 9 kilos of excess weight and his blood sugars by both key measurements are within the "normal range" thus meaning he has reversed the diabetes and is not now diabetic. The so-called experts need to be a lot more open-minded and give very serious considerations to the results which are being obtained. Far too many pontificate with little or no knowledge.'

The forum has with time become a genuine popular democratic uprising animated by the participants' distrust of the conventional medical advice they receive. 'The majority feel the support they receive from their medical professionals and the Health Service in general is either insufficient or inadequate,' notes Dr Roberta Bernardi in an academic survey of 2000 forum members. 'They find the message that diabetes is a progressive disease only to be managed by taking more and more medication to be frustrating and devoid of hope. They desire rather to feel empowered to reverse the condition without the need for medication.'

That empowerment, one of the participants relates, extends to challenging the rationale for other routinely prescribed drugs:

'When the doctor says, "According to the text book ... I want to put you on statins because the recommendation is that all diabetics should have a [cholesterol] level of less than five." Okay, that's nothing to do with me. That is to do with a book that exists in some library somewhere ... it just doesn't feel right, because when you go on the forum you are talking to people who have the same blood glucose as you, the same cholesterol as you ... and so, it feels like a more informed conversation ...'

Stockport family doctor David Unwin, frustrated at the difficulty of controlling his diabetic patients' blood sugar levels, chanced upon the website and, impressed by what he read, persuaded a group of them to 'cut their carbs'. Eight months later they had lost on average a stone (just under 7 kg) in weight, the HbA1c level in all but two was now within the normal range, and they were further rewarded with a fall in both their blood pressure and cholesterol level. His cases included the following:

'A 55-year-old woman presented with tiredness, thirst, an HbA1c of 9.2 per cent and deranged liver function tests caused by a fatty liver. After three months on a low carbohydrate diet her liver tests were normal and HbA1c 6 per cent.

She reported feeling "great, ten years younger" and has lost 7 inches off her waist.'

Commenting on these results, Dr Unwin was 'struck by the energy and enthusiasm of his patients as they took control of their lives instead of waiting for doctors and nurses to solve their problems'. As for the impressive weight loss, he describes how several reported eating considerably less, suggesting their previous high carbohydrate diet 'appeared to be addictive', increasing their appetite – whereas now they 'felt less hungry'.

Dr Unwin's small study could scarcely have been simpler, but that, of course, was precisely the point – for he had demonstrated how a busy family doctor in an urban general practice could make it possible for his diabetic patients to transform their lives for the better in a way that no one had achieved in decades. Anyone could do it, and as the word spread, so they did in their thousands. A popular revolt indeed – fanned, not unreasonably, by a mixture of exultation at how much better they felt and antipathy to the 'so-called experts pontificating with little or no knowledge'.

And so, thirty years after those disastrous 'dietary recommendations' for diabetics in the 1980s, the wheel had turned full circle. 'Carbohydrate restriction is the first approach in diabetes management,' observed Professor Richard Feinman in 2015, citing twelve reasons why it is the better option. They include:

- A raised blood sugar (hyperglycaemia) is the most salient feature of diabetes. Dietary carbohydrate restriction has the greatest effect on decreasing blood glucose levels.
- No dietary intervention is better than carbohydrate restriction for weight loss.

- Patients with Type 2 diabetes on carbohydrate-restricted diets reduce and frequently eliminate the need for medication.
- Glucose lowering by dietary carbohydrate restriction has no side effects comparable to that of pharmacological treatment.

While no one has acknowledged responsibility for the intervening iatrogenic catastrophe, in the same year the British Diabetes Association (now renamed Diabetes UK), sponsor of those 'Dietary recommendations', changed without fanfare the dietary advice on its website from commending 'Five to fourteen portions of starchy foods every day' to 'You may need to restrict your carb intake'.

Epilogue: A master class in deprescribing

Dr Unwin, who as noted above has played an important role in the diabetes counter-revolution, reported the outcome of a consultation with one of his patients, Mr Y, as a 'case history' in the *British Medical Journal*. The summary is as follows:

'Mr Y is a 52-year-old man with a history of type 2 diabetes for fourteen years and hypertension for nine years. He had been experiencing bloating, abdominal pains, and erratic motions for more than a year. He sought advice as to whether any of his other several medical problems might be related to his medication and if he could "cut down on any if they weren't needed".

He was a non-smoker with an alcohol intake of eight units a week. He was taking aspirin 75mg once daily, metformin

500mg three times daily, perindopril (antihypertensive) 4mg daily, and simvastatin 40mg at night.

He weighed 17 stone (steady at this for ten years), his blood pressure was 130/80 mmHg, his glycated haemoglobin (HbA1c) 6.9 per cent and total cholesterol 3.7 mmol/L. His physical examination was normal except for central obesity.

Q: Which of the drugs he is taking would be the most likely to cause his abdominal symptoms?
A: Metformin.

In our clinical practice the most common side effect of metformin is altered bowel habit. Symptoms such as flatulence, nausea, vomiting and abdominal discomfort are common. We know of many patients who have undergone gastrointestinal investigations only to find that their symptoms settled when metformin was withdrawn.

Q: What syndrome does this patient have?
A: The metabolic syndrome.

Hypertension, Type 2 diabetes, central obesity, abnormal liver function tests and dyslipidaemia [raised cholesterol level and triglycerides] are linked by the metabolic syndrome and the common causative factor is obesity. The best remedies are therefore weight loss and exercise.

Q: How could his request to cut down on drugs be handled?
A: Arguably none of his drugs is essential – they have all been prescribed to reduce his risk of cardiovascular

disease and the complications of diabetes, not to treat an actual disease.

Patient outcome:

Mr Y adopted a low carbohydrate diet. He has stopped sugar altogether and cut out bread, potatoes, pasta, cereals and rice. This has led to greater consumption of green vegetables, but also eggs, full fat Greek yoghurt and cheese. He steadily lost a total of 2 stone 7lbs (16 kg) over seven months and successfully stopped all four prescribed drugs, thereby achieving his goal of being medication-free.

His HbA1c is down to 6.1 per cent, blood pressure from 130/80 mmHg to 117/70 mmHg. Both his cholesterol and triglyceride levels have improved.

The weight loss enabled him to take more exercise, join a gym and take up yoga.

His bowel problems and abdominal pains ceased within days of stopping metformin, his energy returned and he now needs an hour and a half less sleep a day.

In general, he reports feeling "just much younger again".'

Chapter 6

Good Doctors and Bad Medicine

'What advice do you have as to how we can resist over-medication by our doctors without antagonising him/her? Quite a number of people I know are fearful of seeing their family doctor because of this. Your guidance would be much appreciated.'

Mrs A. M., Norwich

'Patients come to you and plead, "Please don't give me any tablets – I'll do anything to bring down my blood pressure" even though it is not horrendously high, like, say, 146/90. We have to say to them, "Well, look, we have checked it several times and you're classed as hypertensive. We follow these guidelines and this is what we should be doing with you."'

Practice nurse, 2012

General practice is, for the most part, a fairly humdrum affair – or so it might seem. It does however require a set of sophisticated intellectual skills. They include most notably discernment, the ability almost intuitively to distinguish the serious from the less so and then determine, by asking a few simple questions, which of the dozens of potential reasons why someone might, for example, have a headache or chest pain applies in any individual case. And sympathy too, a genuine understanding of the physical and spiritual misfortunes of being trapped in an unhappy marriage, the burden of caring for dependent elderly relatives, or the futility of being stuck in a dead-end job – and so on – that is the lot of so many. These skills of discernment and sympathy are not given but are rather acquired and refined over time, predicated on the defining feature of general practice, the continuity of the relationship between doctor and patient: 'That shared experience' – which may last for thirty-five years or more of a professional career – notes London family doctor Iona Heath, 'fosters a bond of mutual trust and respect.'

That 'mutual bond of trust and respect' is certainly what people appreciate above all whether it is the friendly informality of the consultation – 'He makes you feel relaxed . . . calls you by your first name, you feel as if you can talk and have a laugh as well which I think is really good . . .'; or whole person 'holistic' care – 'My doctor will say to me "Your mother's got high blood pressure, we'll have to check that next time you come" or whatever, and I like that because they can see patterns in people's lives'; or confidence in the common-sense approach to medical problems – 'If you see a GP you don't know, he can't be sure if you're making it up or exaggerating. I have a sister who has never had anything wrong with her, but is always complaining

"Oh I've got a terrible headache, oh I feel awful." It is not that there's nothing wrong with her, but she moans about it a lot, so I suppose a good GP knows who's like that or who, when saying "I have got a bit of a headache", might actually have meningitis ...'

This almost disingenuous endorsement of the merits, from the patient's perspective, of continuity illustrates its inestimable advantage in interpreting the significance of common symptoms. Her family doctor, aware that her sister is 'always complaining' about her terrible headaches, avoids the major pitfalls of medicine practised out of context such as unnecessary investigations (e.g. costly brain scans) and inappropriate treatment, while attending to the specifics of what might have brought her back to the surgery on this occasion.

There are inevitably those who could tell a different story, frustrated in their dealings with a bored or unsympathetic family doctor. It would, however, have been most unusual, until recently, for anyone such as Mrs A. M. from Norwich cited above to be 'fearful' of seeing her family doctor and to seek advice on how to 'resist over-medication without antagonising him or her'. Her apprehension is well founded given that, as suggested by the practice nurse, 'We follow the guidelines of what we should be doing with you' – i.e. prescribing drugs to lower the blood pressure – even when 'it is not horrendously high'.

The public perception of this shift in the culture of general practice in recent years is illustrated by the following exchange in response to the observation of a reader cited in my medical column: 'We have four permanent GPs in the practice but I no longer know any of them, and no one knows me, apart from what they can glean from the computer screen. Appointments are limited to 7½ minutes – and one quickly becomes conscious of that fact.'

A man, whose father was a GP in the 1950s and 60s, recalled how:

'Besides his morning and evening surgery my father would make about twenty home visits a day. He was also on duty three nights a week and alternate weekends when he was available on the phone, day and night. I am convinced that nowadays GPs would find his workload unbelievable. But he loved his job. And his patients, most of whom he knew well and by name, adored him. Where did it all go wrong?'

Where indeed? This brings us to the third major contributory factor to the rise of polypharmacy – its instrument, as it were: the novel contractual arrangements by which family doctors are now, unlike in the past, financially rewarded for prescribing drugs. No one in their right mind would willingly spend time reading about their GP's method of remuneration and I would not impose on their patience without due cause. So, first a necessary reminder of what is at stake here – the legitimacy (or otherwise) of persuading millions of people they have a potentially life-threatening illness that warrants indefinite drug treatment. Next, the most certain way of 'resisting over-medication' is that they (family doctors) should be aware that you (the reader) know how this situation has come about and their enthusiasm for treating so many is not, as it should be, necessarily driven by concern for their patients' welfare but is also a means for maximising their income.

It all started, seemingly innocently enough, with Prime Minister Tony Blair promising during a television interview in the millennium year 2000 a very substantial increase in funding for the National Health Service – an extra £12 billion over the following six years. His chancellor, Gordon Brown, had not, it subsequently transpired, been consulted on the budgetary implications about which he was understandably less than happy. There were thus no specific plans as to how this financial windfall might be spent, and the wily British Medical Association, the doctors' 'trade union', immediately recognised an opportunity to boost their GP members' earnings. However, this was likely to be tricky. For if GPs were to be paid more they would have to do more, while the priority for many at the time was to do less – to shed their onerous on-call, out-of-surgery-hours commitments at night-time and weekends. Dr Eric Rose, who played an important role in negotiating their contractual arrangements, explains:

'I entered General Practice in 1972 to provide comprehensive care to my patients. I even enjoyed my night calls – especially in the summer – going out and being able to relieve pain or help someone with breathing problems although it didn't stop one from being tired the next day. Over the years, however, things began to change. Most patients are reasonable but an increasing minority came to regard it as their right to call the doctor to visit in the evening regardless of whether it was an emergency. My social life suffered as non-medical friends just couldn't understand why we couldn't join [them for dinner] and even when it was possible, I had a reputation for going to sleep at the table from having been up all night before.'

To be sure, by the late 1990s, the situation Dr Rose describes had certainly improved. GPs organised themselves into 'co-operatives' to provide cover for several practices simultaneously, with an additional £6000 bonus in recognition of their 'out of hours' commitment. For many, however, this could not make up for their disrupted nights and weekends, driving around unfamiliar parts of town (in the days before the marvels of GPS), trying to find an address to which they had been summoned but which perversely never seemed to have the house number prominently displayed.

The challenge, then, for the BMA in obtaining for their GP members a slice of the prime minister's windfall was to come up with a formula that would boost their income over and above the inevitable loss of the bonus from shedding their on-call commitments. The government for their part were understandably not inclined to write a blank cheque that would allow their GPs to carry on as before. Rather they would have to provide objective evidence of their 'increased productivity'. The solution arrived at was that GPs would be 'paid for performance' – for their success in achieving measurable targets of, for example, the proportion of their patients on medication to reduce their blood pressure or cholesterol levels.

And so was born the Quality and Outcomes Framework – a framework (or method) for monitoring – and hopefully improving – the quality and the outcomes of medical interventions. The QOF (pronounced 'quoff'), as it became known, was calibrated according to a points system, whereby GPs could achieve a maximum of 1050 financially rewarded points, 550 of which would be for their endeavours in achieving 76 targets (or indicators) across ten different medical conditions (heart disease, hypertension, diabetes, etc.) – that would make up a quarter of their income. The more points achieved, the higher their earnings would be.

It is impossible to convey in words the scale and complexities of it all, or the profound effects it might have on traditional family doctoring, without reference to what was actually entailed. So, daunting as it might seem, and without the expectation that the reader will scrutinise those initial QOF targets in any detail, Table 6.1 below lists the 12 targets for prevention of heart disease as representative of the 18 for diabetes, 10 for stroke, 5 for hypertension and 8 for lung disease. They would later be considerably expanded.

Table 6.1 QOF clinical indicators: Secondary prevention in coronary heart disease (CHD)

Records	Points
CHD 1. The practice can produce a register of patients with coronary heart disease.	6
Diagnosis and Initial Management	
CHD 2. The percentage of patients with newly diagnosed angina (diagnosed after 1 April 2003) who are referred for exercise testing and/or specialist assessment.	7
Ongoing Management	
CHD 3. The percentage of patients with coronary heart disease whose notes record smoking status in the past 15 months, except those who have never smoked where smoking status need be recorded only once since diagnosis.	7
CHD 4. The percentage of patients with coronary heart disease who smoke, whose notes contain a record that smoking cessation advice or referral to a specialist service, where available, has been offered within the last 15 months.	4
CHD 5. The percentage of patients with coronary heart disease whose notes have a record of blood pressure in the previous 15 months.	7

continued next page ▶

Ongoing Management contd	Points
CHD 6. The percentage of patients with coronary heart disease in whom the last blood pressure reading (measured in the last 15 months) is 150/90 or less.	19
CHD 7. The percentage of patients with coronary heart disease whose notes have a record of total cholesterol in the previous 15 months.	7
CHD 8. The percentage of patients with coronary heart disease whose last measured total cholesterol (measured in last 15 months) is 5mmol/l or less.	16
CHD 9. The percentage of patients with coronary heart disease with a record in the last 15 months that aspirin, an alternative anti-platelet therapy, or an anti-coagulant is being taken (unless a contraindication or side effects are recorded).	7
CHD 10. The percentage of patients with coronary heart disease who are currently treated with a beta blocker (unless a contraindication or side effects are recorded).	7
CHD 11. The percentage of patients with a history of myocardial infarction (diagnosed after 1 April 2003) who are currently treated with an ACE inhibitor or angiotensin II antagonist.	7
CHD 12. The percentage of patients with coronary heart disease who have a record of influenza immunisation in the preceding 1 September to 31 March.	7

From a cursory glance, it will be noted that the first requirement ('Records') is that GPs should keep an updated register of all patients with these various medical conditions. The third step ('ongoing management') – for which, as will be seen, many more 'points' could be earned – requires GPs to ensure that the patients in each category are treated systematically down to the currently accepted definition of 'normal'. This is, as is clear, a formidable undertaking. It requires that all those on the heart disease register, for example, should have a blood pressure of 150/90 or less, a cholesterol level of 5 or less, be taking a beta blocker, an ACE inhibitor, and so on.

This, 'the boldest proposal to improve the quality of General Practice anywhere in the world', according to an editorial in the *British Medical Journal*, would, it was anticipated, abolish the inevitable variability in the quality of the service GPs provided, 'driving up standards' – so the bored or disillusioned or lazy who had previously got away with doing the irreducible minimum would now have to raise their game. Its main selling point, however (and certainly how the BMA sold it to the government), was that it would result in a substantial 'health gain' – for were the benefits of lowering the blood pressure, cholesterol level, etc., as supposed, then the mortality rate from circulatory disorders would tumble – 'saving', it was estimated, 30,000 lives a year.

Furthermore the QOF would also reduce the 'health inequalities' between rich and poor, where the prevalence of heart disease, stroke, etc., is consistently higher in the working compared to the professional classes. It might be reasonable to infer (not necessarily correctly) these inequalities are due to the failure of doctors in deprived areas to adequately address their patients' medical needs. QOF would correct this and, in the long run, would even save the health service money as fewer people would need to be admitted to hospital with coronaries or strokes, complications of their diabetes and so on. So, by paying doctors for their 'performance', everybody would be healthier.

A bold proposal – but also, if inadvertently, the definitive test of the fundamental tenet of the 'population approach', that the mass prescription of statins, antihypertensives, etc., to millions whose physiological measurements might be only marginally above 'normal' offered the greatest opportunity to prevent ill health.

'The profession is being bribed to implement a population-based disease management programme that conflicts with the individual patient-centred ethos of general practice,' observed Newcastle GP Toby Lipman. 'Consequently, the ideal of the "consultation" between doctor and patient as its most important transaction will be undermined by a bureaucratic centralised drive to achieve those targets. The new contract comes close to practising medicine by numbers – and threatens the professional basis of general practice.'

And, enquired Scilly Isles GP Dougal Jeffries, had anyone thought through the implications of what was being asked of them?

'I am increasingly dismayed by the role that has been thrust upon us,' he wrote in the *British Medical Journal*. 'It involves ruthlessly pursuing people who feel perfectly well where the finding of any one of a multitude of minor physiological or biochemical variations can lead to a lifetime of medication, repeated blood tests and other investigations and the adoption of a sickness role that diminishes the overall quality of life. I prefer the idea of seeing patients who are actually ill rather than those whom epidemiologists and pharmaceutical companies believe to be in need of drug treatment.'

Still, most GPs were in favour. To be sure, QOF would complicate their lives enormously but making it work also offered a novel intellectual challenge. It might seem a bureaucratic nightmare, but computer systems would handle the prodigious amount of data they now had to collect while much of the hard graft could be delegated to others. Then it could be argued that QOF provided a definitive structure around which they could organise the management of their patients with chronic illnesses. And, frabjous joy, they were now no longer, as before, expected to be responsible for their patients' welfare around the clock, 365 days a year. The loss of the £6000 bonus from their on-call commitment would be more than made up for from Prime Minister Tony Blair's extra funding, of which they were allocated a generous slice of £1 billion a year. Their BMA negotiators had done them proud. In 2004 more than three-quarters voted in favour of the new contract. A sensible decision as it turned out – for, thanks to the QOF, their earnings would rise by 50 per cent to a generous £113,614 a year for a partner – a tidy sum for a now reasonable working week of around fifty hours.

Four years on, in 2008 the QOF was more than up and running; indeed GPs had surpassed themselves. The new contract, costed in anticipation that they would achieve 75 per cent of the points available, had seriously underestimated their organisational skills as they routinely hit 90 per cent or more – for which the Treasury then had to pay out almost half as much again (£400 million) over and above the original £1 billion allocated to the scheme. The Department of Health, embarrassed at having been so thoroughly outmanoeuvred by the wily BMA – and by stories in the press of doctors now being paid so much more for working fewer hours – responded by tightening the screw, with a host of new 'targets' they would have to reach. They were now required to interrogate their patients to see whether they might be suffering from depression or have early signs of dementia, test their kidney function, treat disturbances of heart rhythm more vigorously and – a powerful engine of medicalisation – calculate everyone's coronary risk score, the obscure statistical algorithm that ostensibly predicts the risk of a future coronary.

Many seemed not unduly concerned by the transition from their previous status as 'independent contractors', now compelled to jump through an ever-escalating number of hoops to hit those government-imposed targets. There was professional satisfaction in the obvious improvement in their 'performance' – with a sharp increase, by over a quarter, in the numbers of their patients diagnosed as having diabetes (an additional 250,000 in England alone) and with one in four of adults now identified as having raised blood pressure. Satisfaction too in their patients being so much better (or more thoroughly) treated, their blood pressure and glucose levels reduced to below those target thresholds of 'normal'. 'The QOF is just an additional motivation to make sure we are practising good medicine,' observed one of a dozen GPs responding to a survey on the impact of the financial incentives. 'Overall it's good and I think the fact that we are getting new targets is really important. So I am quite positive about it really.'

Another was not so sanguine: 'There is more of an emphasis on gathering information than caring for the patient. I get frustrated with QOF targets for they treat a patient not as the person they really are but as a condition.' Citing the example of being required to prescribe statins to a 92-year-old woman, he asked, 'If it's actually not pertinent to the person sitting in front of you, what am I doing this for? That becomes number crunching, ticking boxes.'

The essential problem, hinted at here, was that the more successful GPs were in hitting their targets, and the more targets there were to hit, the more apparent the constraints on their professional judgement of what might be appropriate in any clinical situation. Whereas there had always been just two people, the doctor and patient, in the consulting room, now there was a third intrusive voice to which the doctor had to pay heed. Thus, there are any number of things one might wish to discuss with a 92-year-old woman, both medical (how are the knees?) and more general (how are the grandchildren?). But, the moment the GP turned to his computer screen, the third voice would intrude with a reminder to test her cholesterol level, thus hijacking the flow of the conversation about knees and grandchildren in favour of why, at her age, she needed to take cholesterol-lowering statins.

There were, after all, no points to be earned from enquiring after the knees or the grandchildren, or taking a detailed history to make sense of some puzzling symptom, or indeed any of the traditional skills of family doctoring – all of which can take time. But time is limited and though GPs might claim, naturally enough, that QOF had not changed the nature of their own practice, they knew of others for whom it had. 'The practices that are more organised in terms of getting the QOF points go bish-bang-wallop through the scoring. They say "We won't do that because it's not a QOF thing, we're not going to bother with it."'

And those motivated by financial incentives to 'bish-bang-wallop through the scoring' might also be incentivised to 'game the system'. Let's be slightly sceptical for a moment about GPs' impressive performance in hitting all those targets, thus maximising their income by obtaining a near optimum number of points. Why was it, wondered Welsh GP Dr Jonathan Richards, that his fellow doctors in other general practices should be doing so much better than he was at hitting the target for the number of his patients with well-controlled blood pressure? Every time he measured someone's blood pressure he entered the reading into the computer records. Were other GPs doing the same or were they entering the required rather than the true reading?

'When it comes to making the computer entry of a blood pressure reading,' he asks, 'where are the lines between accuracy, probity, game-playing, cheating and fraud? Mrs Jones's systolic blood pressure reading is above the target value. If it is 151mmHg (millimetres of mercury) can I enter 150 into the records with a clear conscience since everyone knows that the machines are not that accurate? If 151 can become 150, what about 152, 153 or 154? How many millimetres of mercury matter clinically, how many ethically, and how many financially?'

And Dr Richards draws attention to another 'gaming' wheeze. GPs are permitted under the new contract to exclude patients from their QOF calculations if, for example, despite much badgering they refuse to attend the surgery to have their blood pressure measured. This is known as 'exception reporting'. So, let's say there are several patients in your practice whose blood pressure is proving difficult to control, posing a serious obstacle to hitting the target for the proportion successfully treated. It is then very much in your financial interest to 'exception report' them (giving some spurious reason) so they don't bring down your QOF score, while boosting the numbers on the register whose blood pressure is only marginally above the threshold and thus more likely to rapidly come within target level. A Scottish GP explains:

'We gain £1800 by omitting 110 poorly controlled patients and recording 110 well controlled patients. This is clearly an incentive to target a practice's limited resources towards frequent recall and measurement of well controlled patients rather than the time-consuming and difficult task of improving those whose blood pressure is poorly controlled.'

Massaging the figures may perhaps not be that important, though one might worry about its insidious effect on doctors' moral values. More serious are the financial inducements to practise bad medicine. Consider Mrs Smith, a new patient, middle-aged and a bit overweight. You have just taken her blood pressure, which is slightly raised at 160/100. What do you do? You could ensure it really is elevated by taking it several times and, if it is, discuss 'lifestyle changes' such as losing a few pounds and taking more exercise, which might help bring it down – and arrange to review the situation in a couple of months' time. She may by then have heeded your advice, lost some weight so her blood pressure now falls within the normal range. It is however much more sensible, if the GP is to maximise his income, to start her on the pills immediately. These are guaranteed to bring her blood pressure down and take him one step nearer to his target of the proportion of patients with well-controlled hypertension. Thus good doctors end up practising bad medicine.

'The QOF is deeply corrosive of the ethical practice of medicine,' lamented Professor Dee Mangin of McMaster University, Ontario, in a much-cited commentary in the *British Journal of General Practice*:

'This disempowering, if well paid, system of micro-management focused on measurable indicators [is the antithesis] of what people value: trust, reassurance and the appreciation of context. It incentivises (coerces) GPs to persuade patients to take medicines in return for financial gain, [a situation] no different in principle from taking payments from a pharmaceutical company for prescribing a particular drug. It could only lead to a loss of critical thinking, de-professionalisation and a loss of respect for the autonomy of doctors.'

Still, the QOF, being 'Quite Obviously Flawed', she noted, was at least appropriately named.

Two months later, a couple of epidemiologists – whose discipline had done so much to promote the cause of mass medication – broke ranks in an article, 'Measuring performance but missing the point'. Here they drew attention to the deception involved in supposing GPs were being financially rewarded for 'quality and outcomes'. To be sure they might be surpassing themselves, indeed over-performing, in achieving all those 'points', but the 'point' of medicine, the only quality outcome that matters, is whether the patient benefits.

'None of the framework's measures estimate clinically important outcomes,' they noted. 'What they assess rather is processes (such as lowering blood pressure and cholesterol levels) that are presumed to lead to better outcomes. But until it can be shown these translate into tangible improvements (such as fewer hospital admissions, lower mortality rates, etc.), the true benefits and cost-effectiveness of the QOF cannot be estimated.'

Hang on a minute, responded Martin Roland, a professor of general practice and one of the main architects of the QOF: 'Many GPs are strong supporters of a system that they believe has helped them to deliver high quality care. Some believe it has given them more time with patients, with routine tasks delegated to others.' To be sure it was necessary to minimise the potential harms, and 'If it becomes clear that QOF is having a damaging effect we should argue for a reduction in its contribution to GP income in future years.'

This, however, would result in a substantial loss of earnings, and so was unlikely to happen. Anyhow, the genie was out of the bottle. The government had established a system for directly controlling what GPs did and now they must dance to its tune.

Meanwhile, what did the public make of all this? They were unlikely to be enthusiastic about their doctors now being 'paid for performance' – had they known about it. But there were no notices or leaflets in the surgery informing them of these changes in their doctors' contractual arrangements. 'I have asked many people over the years whether they have heard of the QOF,' observes Charlotte Williamson, chair of the Patient Liaison Group at the Royal College of General Practitioners. 'Few have. All were surprised and dismayed when I outlined the financial inducements.'

That silence might be described as deafening. None of those interviewed in a patient survey in 2012 – eight years after the introduction of the QOF – were aware of the radical change in GPs' methods of remuneration. Once informed, most thought it 'inappropriate'.

'I certainly didn't realise that they got an extra payment for taking somebody's blood pressure, good heavens. Personally, I think it's wrong. Doctors should deliver [a high] quality of care because it's the professional thing to do.'

'You would like to think they were doing what they felt to be necessary rather than possibly, oh well, if we do this we get extra pay. I don't like the idea of that.'

And they readily appreciated how it could be detrimental to 'holistic' care:

'I know what it's like to be orientated to hitting targets, you ignore other important issues. The doctor may have ticked a box that he has prescribed x amount of medication – but it is not necessarily the treatment that is most appropriate.'

Doctors could rationalise their reticence about the new arrangements on the grounds that scepticism about those financial incentives (had their patients known about them) might prompt awkward questions as to whether they really needed the drugs being prescribed. This seems in retrospect a collective, if understandable, exercise in self-deception, a defence mechanism against acknowledging the degree to which the QOF compromised their professional and clinical standards. Inevitably, inescapably, the pursuit of the QOF targets redefined their relationship with their patients, who now became, as one GP expressed it bluntly, 'walking bags of money' – monetarised commodities whose worth could only be realised by measuring their cholesterol levels and prescribing pills. Lots of pills.

Surely not – but tragically only too true, as revealed by a fly-on-the-wall study from Durham University investigating the practicalities of how QOF's monetary logic had come to distort medical priorities. The following exchange is illustrative:

'GP: Hmm ... you know, there are some we get a lot more for and some we don't get much at all ... so £12? I wouldn't worry about that; £37 ... hmm? (hesitating) ... you know it's in their hundreds that we should be looking at ... £770 ... and that's only three patients ...
Researcher: So, three patients are worth more than ...
GP: £259 per patient, if I can get those three ...

Researcher: How do they decide this condition is worth more than the others?
GP: I have no idea ...'

Or again, another GP explains to colleagues how to work the system ('I'm bragging, I can make £4000 in one session'):

'There's not many things in QOF where your limited number of patients buys you so many points; and I have managed to pick up lots of ones like ... cardiovascular. So ... my time so far has been really good value ... and I have picked up the learning disability ... the Down's syndrome ... we've got one patient and he's worth ... three points, etc., etc.'

Then a GP describes the 'nightmare' of the drive to hit targets towards the end of the financial year:

'There's osteoporosis, we haven't hit it [yet], diabetes, we've only got three points [out of thirteen] so we haven't hit it; we need 130 patients for blood pressure ... but we need 211 urine tests, to get the money or otherwise we don't get it!'

This frenetic activity, it might be noted, illustrates the QOF's two main injurious consequences – besides, of course, over-treatment. First is the mismatch of priorities: the patient's that the particular problem he brings to the doctor will be sorted out is quite different from the doctor's whose efforts are directed to ensuring the tasks and laboratory tests necessary to achieve those targets have been achieved. And it is also, at least potentially, damaging to the 'holistic' nature of the clinical encounter between the doctor and his patients as individuals, reducing them to so many remunerative bio-markers (cholesterol, blood pressure level, etc.) or diagnostic categories (osteoporosis, diabetes, etc.).

It also inevitably entails a degree of subterfuge to conceal, under the guise of beneficence, the financial incentives behind all these medical interventions. We have already encountered this in the opening chapter, in the innocent invitation for a flu jab, a covert means of enticing the unwary into the surgery to institute that income-generating regime for treating their 'raised' blood pressure.

To be sure, doctors may rationalise this subterfuge as a means of identifying those who might require treatment. But it also discourages an open discussion about the genuine risks associated with what for most are marginally raised physiological variables – and the modest benefits of medication.

Then inducing unnecessary alarm in patients should be the antithesis of good doctoring, one of whose primary tasks is to reassure the apprehensive. It is, however, an endemic feature of the QOF, burdening many with the anxiety of being wrongly labelled as having not just 'raised cholesterol' but even dementia or chronic kidney disease.

Dementia is, for obvious reasons, probably the most feared diagnosis of all. It is quite distinct from what is known as mild cognitive impairment (MCI) – forgetfulness, difficulty in recalling names, and so on – which is the lot of virtually every-one in their seventies and beyond. To be sure, around 5 per cent of those with MCI will go on to develop true dementia, but it is impossible to determine who they might be – nor is there any point in doing so, as there is no specific treatment. In 2006 the government introduced a new QOF target intended to boost the numbers so diagnosed, paying GPs a bonus of £55 for subjecting their patients to a psychological questionnaire with a series of cognitive tests that ostensibly could identify dementia in its early stages. This too required GPs to resort to subterfuge to claim their fee – as an 81-year-old man describes:

'Completely out of the blue I had a phone call asking me to attend the surgery to have my blood pressure taken. I was rather bemused, what with the trauma in the last year of having had a cancer operation and radiotherapy, but attended nonetheless. After the BP test the doctor asked me to draw a clock face in a circle on a sheet of paper. I asked if this were a dementia test and she declined to reply. Other memory and cognitive tests followed, e.g. a random name and address, reciting numbers backwards, etc. I asked if she could recite the alphabet backwards (as I can at speed) but she declined. In retrospect, I felt I should have walked out. The invitation to have my blood pressure measured was so blatantly a devious ruse to get me to the surgery. And when she refused to confirm what the cognitive tests were for, that was so rude. I felt I was being treated like an ignorant "specimen" to fulfil the practice quota.'

His closing sentence, some might think, is particularly poignant:

'I felt like writing a strong letter of complaint but desisted as I was fearful that, if I rubbed them up the wrong way, it would make things difficult when I really needed their help.'

There was, needless to say, no attempt to spell out the poor discriminatory power of this psychometric inquisition that, given to a hundred people, will misdiagnose dementia in twenty-three of them. But, as the wife of another 81-year-old who initially 'failed' the psychometric test found, it verged on the farcical – though not before having a devastating effect on his morale:

'The last time my husband visited the surgery, the practice nurse asked him to remember a name before asking a couple of questions – one of which was to name the medication he takes. As neither he nor I can pronounce them, let alone remember the names, this seemed a little futile. What does it matter anyway? He keeps his medicines in two plastic bags – one for the morning and one for the evening – and takes them appropriately. After he was unable to tell her the names of his medication, she then asked him for the name he had been asked to remember. By this time, and a bit confused, he had no idea – so he was told he had "borderline" dementia.

Since then, he sees everything as evidence of a slide into senility where forgetting the name of somebody/something is part-way towards the end and he is terrified that he will shortly be dragged off to a nursing home. It has been an uphill struggle to reassure him that nothing of the sort will take place and that nodding off of an afternoon or forgetting names and places is quite normal at his age. He visited the surgery yesterday by which time he had committed his medicines to memory. He was asked the self-same questions and passed 100 per cent. So what use are these questions when all they do is frighten people into thinking they are in decline which can so often lead to just that . . .'

This thoughtless harm from conflating – for a very modest financial gain – a natural age-determined fall-off in mental acuity with a dread disease is apparent too in those labelled as having 'chronic kidney disease'. The physiological capacity of the kidneys to filter out the waste products of metabolism, such as urea, is far in excess of that required for normal functioning. It is, after all, possible to get by just as well with one kidney as with two. So, while for many of those in their seventies and beyond the kidneys' 'filtration rate' will be lower than when in their twenties, it is more than enough to see them out. But then the experts decreed that those in whom the filtration rate was half or less than 'normal' should be labelled as having chronic kidney disease – and again, GPs were financially rewarded for the numbers of patients so diagnosed.

By this criterion, nearly half of those over the age of seventy-five have this condition – almost two million people – for just 1700 of whom it will be a meaningful diagnosis indicating poor functioning of the kidneys of such severity as to warrant dialysis or transplantation. There is, of course, no reason why the 1,998,000 misleadingly labelled as having 'chronic kidney disease' should be aware of this; rather, reasonably enough, they are likely to assume that though they might feel healthy, their kidneys are in a bad way and it is only a matter of time before they need to be hooked up to a dialysis machine. And that, indeed, is just what happens, as another GP describes:

'They come to the surgery because they are feeling tired or for investigation of anaemia or all sorts of other things. And so, you measure that filtration rate which turns out to be below the threshold for "chronic kidney disease". Then there is lots of confusion. Many think they would need to have dialysis in a couple of years' time. So, there is a lot of anxiety. You need to explain in some detail "what does chronic kidney disease actually mean?"'

It 'means', of course, nothing. Chronic kidney disease is not a 'disease' at all but a physiological measurement of kidney function, repurposed as a remunerated QOF target. Its potential to generate unwarranted anxiety is, as for those wrongly labelled as having dementia, considerable. A seventy-year-old woman describes her experience:

'To be honest, it did scare me. You hear the words "kidney disease" and immediately think of dialysis. I did feel better when I was told it was probably just part of getting older but I went on the internet when I got home and everything you read there scares you. A few months later I felt better – my GP didn't seem too worried about it and hadn't given me any medication so it couldn't be that bad. I think it's the word "chronic" that's most worrying. It makes you feel like you're just going to fade away and I did think, is this going to be the start of me being really ill?'

These two QOF targets were clearly indefensible. The dementia target was eventually dropped and that for chronic kidney disease much modified. But the principle of GPs being 'paid for performance' endures, with all its potential to coarsen the clinical encounter, subvert the bond of trust and promote polypharmacy. Still, for all that, perhaps ultimately it has been in a good cause. Almost fifteen years have elapsed since the launch of 'this boldest proposal to improve the quality of General Practice anywhere in the world', time enough for a reasonable verdict as to whether it has reduced the toll of strokes and heart disease or improved the quality of care of those with, for example, diabetes. At an estimated cost of £1.5 billion a year it certainly should have, but if it has not this is a matter of the utmost importance. For the QOF, as noted, is the definitive test of that immensely influential 'population approach', the necessity for treating millions in anticipation of benefit to a few.

We shall start with the most frequently cited evidence in favour of the QOF: its role in improving the quality of care for the millions with diabetes through a more systematic approach to its treatment and the prevention of complications. Then we shall turn to the 'bottom line', the crucial question posed by the dissident epidemiologists in their article 'Measuring performance but missing the point' – has the QOF significantly ameliorated the burden of illness and improved everyone's health?

Diabetes

'Maturity onset' or Type 2 diabetes is the jewel in the crown of the QOF system, with more financially incentivised targets (seventeen), generating more income (£12,700), than any other condition. There is thus every reason for doctors to diagnose as many cases as possible; and, as already noted, within three years they had identified an impressive 250,000 new cases. The 'real-isation' of the worth to the practice of all those on the diabetes register was a formidable task, requiring – if those seventeen targets were to be achieved – a systematic approach of annual check-ups and blood tests to monitor not just the blood sugar but all those potential complications outlined in the previous chapter: the 'macrovascular': heart disease, strokes and poor circulation; and 'microvascular': its adverse effects on the functioning of the eyes, kidneys, nerves and so on.

Their efforts could scarcely have been more successful. There was a quantum leap in the proportion of patients in whom these indicators were routinely measured and who were placed on appropriate medication, from less than half prior to the initiation of the QOF to more than 90 per cent. Many no doubt benefited but a substantial proportion did not, starting with those whose modestly raised blood sugar was readily reversible with simple dietary measures. We have already considered in the previous chapter how the near doubling of the numbers with diabetes over the past thirty years (up from 1.8 million to more than 3 million) is in large part an iatrogenic catastrophe fuelled by the perverse advocacy of that high carbohydrate/low fat diet that promotes obesity and increases the need for medication to lower the blood sugar level. The pursuit of those QOF targets would have accelerated this process (how many of those 250,000 additional cases did indeed have diabetes?) while turning up the volume of medicalisation.

Diabetes, no matter how mild or indeed reversible, it was emphasised, was a 'lifelong condition' requiring constant surveillance – once trapped in the web of its annual blood test and examinations there could be no escape. 'It was all something of a shock,' begins a familiar story:

'Following a routine blood test I received a letter from my GP's practice advising me I had a "slightly raised blood sugar level" and was called in for a follow-up test. The doctor welcomed me with the words that I had Type 2 diabetes, the normal causes of which were "overweight, lack of exercise and unhealthy diet". Why, asked my wife, should this affect me, given I was not overweight, took plenty of exercise and was very diet conscious? Looking at her and ignoring me, he said, "Let's face it, your husband is seventy-three, his organs are slowly conking out – and my job is to keep him ticking over." I was handed over to the hawkish attention of the diabetes nurse, who insisted that there was no such thing as "marginal" diabetes:

like pregnancy, one either is or one isn't. I was – and would be carefully monitored for the rest of my life.'

The suspicion that labelling those with a marginally raised blood sugar as diabetic – even if the level subsequently reverted to normal – might be a ruse to boost family doctors' income is echoed by a self-styled 'victim' of what he describes as the 'Diabetes Taliban':

'Four years ago, I went to my GP for a routine appointment following a knee replacement when, without warning, he insisted on taking blood to check for diabetes. This was despite my telling him that I had only just finished breakfast. Two days later he called to tell me my blood sugar was over the limit, albeit not by much, and that I was diabetic. Due to inactivity before and after my knee operation I had put on a few pounds. I was intending to diet anyway so I cut back on carbohydrates and sugar for a few months and lost the unwanted weight. Since then I have reverted to my previous diet, not put the weight back on and my blood sugar readings have never exceeded the limits. When I asked my doctor whether I really am diabetic he said that once a diabetic, always a diabetic but, in my case, it is mild. I don't believe him but I am not prepared to argue, though it is inconvenient to have to declare a condition which I don't believe I suffer from every time I go for medical or dental treatment. The real problem for me, however, is that I am aware his practice income is to some extent dependent on how many people he identifies as suffering from one of a prescribed list of conditions. As I have told him, in my view, this both undermines the traditional doctor/patient relationship and is unethical.'

Meanwhile, as also described in the previous chapter, the pursuit of the target of 'tight control', reducing with a combination of diabetes drugs the blood sugar to the 'threshold' level of 7.5 mmol/L or less, did not, as had been hoped for, significantly reduce the risk of heart attacks and strokes or 'microvascular complications'. It did, however, predispose to the major hazard of over-treatment – excess lowering of the blood sugar (or hypoglycaemia) warranting medical intervention to correct it. It was a similar story with the cholesterol-lowering statins, their universal prescription a further QOF target for all those with diabetes but which, unhappily for some, has the side effect of increasing their blood sugar level and thus their further need for medication.

The verdict on the 'jewel in the crown' of the QOF system, then, might seem equivocal. The 90 per cent success rate in hitting those targets was certainly most impressive, to the advantage no doubt of many, but at the cost of over-diagnosis, over-treatment, polypharmacy, iatrogenic illness and remorseless medicalisation, where even those with marginally raised glucose levels were subjected to a regime of intense medical surveillance.

The bottom line

And so, finally, to the bottom line of this vastly ambitious venture of paying doctors for their performance conducted without the knowledge or consent of its millions of unwitting participants. The total cost over the past fifteen years is in the region of £25–£30 billion – £15 billion in direct payments to general practitioners and a similar sum for the polypharmacy it has generated: a doubling or more of the number of prescriptions for statins, blood pressure-lowering medication and diabetes drugs, 60 per cent more antidepressants, and so on. So, a lot of money that would perhaps have been spent to better advantage in some other way – building, for example, a thousand brand-new hospitals, or providing free residential care to all with dementia. Then there are the hidden 'opportunity' costs of the time spent by family doctors administering the QOF that could have been spent more productively – and the hidden, unmeasured iatrogenic costs of polypharmacy.

The prospectus on which the BMA back in 2004 had sold the new GP contract to the government would have seemed, at the time, very attractive – allowing politicians to take the credit for the anticipated tumbling rates of stroke and heart disease, the narrowing of health inequalities between rich and poor and the prolongation of life expectancy, 'saving' an estimated 30,000 lives a year. More than a decade later, it is possible to assess the progress made in achieving those very desirable goals. The number of referrals and admissions to hospitals certainly should have fallen but, on the contrary, throughout this period they have continued to rise at a rate of 5 per cent per year, though those for heart disease have been slightly lower than the trend would predict. Next, the health gap between the social classes: the QOF, as has been noted, certainly 'drove up standards', with near uniform success in hitting those targets throughout the country – but this has had no demonstrable influence on the persistent discrepancy in health between the better and less well off. Finally, the prospect of saving 30,000 lives a year has proved to be a mirage, with a review of the relevant evidence concluding: 'Our results show the introduction of the QOF was not associated with significant changes in mortality for the diseases targeted by the programme.'

To summarise, according to a government-sponsored Review of the Quality and Outcome Framework, published in 2016: 'We have found no definitive evidence that QOF has had any significant effect on emergency admissions or population health or that it is an effective method for reducing inequalities in health and healthcare.'

It is impossible to over-emphasise the significance of this conclusion as the definitive refutation of the bizarre doctrine (as now it seems) promoted by Geoffrey Rose and those influential epidemiologists – that the 'population is sick', their 'normal' physiological variables in fact 'abnormal', warranting medication to lower them. From this perspective the £25–£30 billion cost of the QOF has, one might argue, actually been money well spent. The most expensive, albeit unintentional, experiment in the history of medicine certainly – but its verdict on the putative benefits of mass medicalisation could not be more unequivocal. So the population was not 'sick' after all, but it has certainly been made 'sick' by the consequences of profligate over-prescribing – resulting, as will be seen in the next chapter, almost certainly in shortened lives for many.

'The QOF simply hasn't worked,' observed Glasgow GP Des Spence, writing in the *British Medical Journal* in 2014. 'It is a bureaucratic disaster, measuring the measurable but eroding the all-important immeasurable, and squandering our time, efforts and money. It has made patients of us all and turned skilled clinicians into bean counters. It's time to look away from the computer screen and at the patient once again. Turn off the financial life support and let this failed intervention die.'

Epilogue: Ten commandments

The perverse incentives for good doctors to practise bad medicine prompted a group of general practitioners to draw up the following ten commandments. They are, in light of the above, self-explanatory.

1. Thou shalt have no aim except to help patients according to the goals they wish to achieve.
2. Thou shalt always seek knowledge of the benefits, harms and costs of treatment, and share this knowledge at all times.
3. Thou shalt, if all else fails, or if the evidence is lacking, happily consider watchful waiting as an appropriate course of action.
4. Thou shalt honour balanced sources of knowledge, and keep thyself from all who seek to deceive thee.
5. Thou shalt treat according to level of risk and not to level of risk factor.
6. Thou shalt not bow down to treatment targets designed by committees for these are but graven images.
7. Honour thy older patients, for although they often have the highest risk, they also have the highest risk of harm from treatment.
8. Thou shalt stop any treatment that is not of clear benefit.
9. Thou shalt diligently try to find the best treatment for the individual because different treatments suit different people.
10. Thou shalt seek to use as few drugs as possible.

Chapter 7

Oldies – The Great Betrayal

*Drug therapy in the elderly should be kept
to a minimum*

D. R. Laurence,
Clinical Pharmacology, 1987

Those in their seventies and beyond are, by far, the major beneficiaries of modern medicine. Every year tens of thousands previously doomed to blindness from cataracts, immobility from crippling arthritis, and crushing chest pains from angina have their lives transformed by the staggeringly successful procedures of, respectively, an intraocular lens implant, joint replacement or coronary angioplasty. And so too with those immensely useful and effective drugs – steroids, anti-inflammatories, acid suppressants, diuretics, muscle relaxants, antidepressants and so on – that vanquish (or mitigate) the trials and tribulations of later life: muscular aches and pains, arthritic joints, heartburn from acid reflux, heart failure, low mood and so on. Many, troubled by more than one of these symptoms, will need to take a combination of appropriate medications. Here, polypharmacy is an inevitable (and indispensable) feature of ageing and to be welcomed. But caution is necessary. 'Any drug that is worth using can cause harm,' notes Emeritus Professor D. R. Laurence in the introduction to his classic textbook *Clinical Pharmacology* – required reading for medical students for many years – and after considering the eight reasons for their increased tendency to cause harm in later life, he asserts the unassailable conclusion that 'Drug therapy in the elderly should be kept to a minimum'.

Here we examine in this book's penultimate and – in practical terms – most important chapter how, over the past decades, this cardinal rule of prescribing has been wilfully ignored and the serious consequences for so many. The betrayal of the trust older patients place in their doctors that they will not burden them with unnecessary medication is encapsulated in the following four citations. We start with the 'Rising Tide of Polypharmacy':

'Between 1995 and 2010 the proportion of adults dispensed more than five drugs doubled to 20% and the proportion dispensed more than ten tripled to 6%. The prescription of more than ten drugs was strongly associated with increasing age. The proportion of potentially serious drug–drug interactions more than doubled.

Conclusion: Drug regimes are increasingly complex and potentially harmful.'

Bruce Guthrie et al., 'The Rising Tide of Polypharmacy', *BMC Medicine* (2015)

Next, we find, this 'rising tide of polypharmacy' is correlated with an increasing number of diagnoses. This could be because doctors are more thorough in investigating their elderly patients than in the past and are thus discovering more treatable conditions. Alternatively, it could be that the previously 'normal' for this age group is now deemed to be 'abnormal', thus warranting treatment:

'There were major increases in recorded prevalence of most conditions. In the eighty-five plus age group the proportion with more than three rose from 32% to 55% and the proportion taking more than three drugs rose from 45% to 66%. The proportion with more than one hospital admission a year rose from 28% to 65%.

Conclusion: There has been a dramatic increase in the medicalisation of the old evidenced in increased diagnosis, prescribing and hospitalisation.'

David Melzer, 'Much more medicine for the oldest old', *Age and Ageing* (2014)

'The rising tide of polypharmacy' is, too, inevitably associated with more serious adverse reactions warranting admission to hospital, though the scale and the resulting fatal outcomes may seem shocking:

'Between 1999 and 2008 the annual hospital admissions due to adverse drug reactions increased by 76.8% and the in-hospital mortality rate by 10%. There has been a near two-fold increase in nephropathy (kidney damage) and cardiovascular consequences due to drugs.

Conclusion: The number of admissions due to adverse drug

reactions has increased at a greater rate than the increase in total hospital admissions.'

Tai-yin Wu, 'Ten-year trends in hospital admissions for adverse drug reactions in England, 1999–2009', *Journal of the Royal Society of Medicine* (2010)

Finally, Nigel Hawkes, formerly science correspondent for *The Times*, reflects on the 'sensational' sharp increase in mortality rates in the older age group which, in the light of the above, is almost certainly related to over-prescribing:

'The figures are fairly sensational given the long experience of steadily rising life expectancy. Starting in 2012, deaths have been consistently higher, and by strikingly larger margins than they were in the years 2008 to 2011. There are sharp increases in the older age groups, especially marked in those aged over sixty-five. Averaged over the first twenty-six weeks of 2013 there have been about ten thousand five hundred deaths a week, which is roughly six hundred more than would have been expected – a 5.6% increase. That is enormous.'

Nigel Hawkes, 'The curious case of six hundred extra deaths a week', *British Medical Journal* (2013)

This rising incidence of drug-induced hospital admissions and the 'sensational' sharp increase in mortality rates can only be an indicator of the much wider problem of iatrogenic illness.

The following letter from a woman whose 71-year-old husband is taking eight pills in the morning, five in the evening speaks for itself:

'My husband has lost all confidence. He gets up in the morning with no energy and this continues all day long, he is not able to work in the house or the garden. He occasionally washes the dishes but this is too much for him. When our grandchildren visit it is all too much for him which is sad. His life stretches out with no hope for improvement. On enquiring about the necessity for taking so many medications, the GP said that he would not be here if he stopped any of them.'

That closing observation takes us, as will be seen, to the heart of the problem of polypharmacy in the elderly.

The corollary of the above is obvious enough. There can be no more predictably beneficial 'treatment' for those in their seventies and beyond than to reduce the number of drugs they are taking, as this might be expected to simultaneously alleviate their iatrogenic symptoms, reduce their risk of requiring admission to hospital and prolong their lives. A felicitous outcome indeed, demonstrated unequivocally a decade ago when Israeli physician Dr Doron Garfinkel discontinued 320 drugs (nitrates, acid suppressants, antihypertensives, diuretics, etc.) in more than a hundred frail nursing-home residents. Over the following year, when compared to a 'controlled group', the numbers dying fell from 45 per cent to 21 per cent and those requiring emergency admission to hospital from 30 per cent to 11 per cent. This is a better result than that achieved by any drug treatment, ever, anywhere. Three years later he repeated the exercise in patients living at home, 88 per cent of whom reported feeling physically and mentally much improved. From this, Dr Garfinkel concluded that polypharmacy should, on its own account, be conceived as a disease 'with potentially more complications than the illnesses these different drugs are prescribed for'.

So why do doctors not follow Dr Garfinkel's good example? It is not as if they fail to acknowledge the problem – in a poll of those attending a GP conference in London in 2014, nine out of ten conceded they were over-treating their older patients. A year later, the delegates at the annual conference of the Royal College of General Practitioners examined the issue during a session with the provocative title 'My Doctor makes me sick. What can we do about it?' – the proposed 'solution' being that GPs be financially rewarded for their success in 'deprescribing', reducing the number of drugs their older patients were taking.

For all that, the over-medicalisation of oldies remains as prevalent as ever. There would seem no alternative for those seeking to protect themselves, or their parents or older relatives, against those iatrogenic harms than to have some understanding of the reasons behind the inversion of Professor Laurence's wise dictum, the necessity of 'keeping drug therapy in the elderly to a minimum'.

* * *

The prevalence of adverse effects in oldies is three times higher than for the relatively young, from which one might infer drugs are intrinsically more dangerous. Professor Laurence lists eight 'contributing factors' that fall into two broad categories. The first concerns the action of a drug in the body, or pharmacokinesis. Drugs exert their therapeutic effect by influencing the chemistry of the body, which depends on their 'concentration', i.e. the amount circulating in the blood: too little and the drug is ineffective, too much and it can be harmful. That concentration in turn will depend on the distribution of the drug between the compartments of the body, its detoxification in the liver and its elimination through the kidneys. Each of these three aspects of pharmacokinesis becomes less efficient with age. So, for example, impaired functioning of the liver (metabolism) or kidney (excretion) may increase the concentration of a drug in the blood and tissues to potentially dangerous levels.

The second category of factors increasing the vulnerability of oldies to adverse effects concerns the influence of ageing on the miracle of homeostasis, the myriad of physiological processes ensuring that, moment by moment for decades on end, the levels of the thousands of proteins and chemicals in the body remain within the same narrow limits necessary for their proper functioning. Thus, it does not matter whether your last meal was five minutes, five hours or five days ago, the amount of the energy-producing fuel glucose in the blood hardly alters. These homeostatic mechanisms that maintain the constancy of the 'milieu intérieur' (as it is known) also become less efficient with age, and thus the elderly are less able to make the necessary adjustments that will, for example, counter the drop in blood pressure on standing that may be induced by blood pressure-lowering medication. Put simply, oldies are less equipped to 'handle' the drugs they take and accommodate their untoward physiological effects.

That apart, there is a long list of drugs that are generally considered 'unsafe' or 'should be avoided' or are 'specifically contra-indicated' but which, as no doctor could conceivably know the ramifications of each and every one, are nonetheless routinely prescribed. Thus, an investigation of the factors contributing to the hospital admission of 2000 patients found they were, on average, each taking seven drugs; for two-thirds of them this included at least one 'inappropriate medication', resulting in an adverse drug reaction in one-fifth. Then, the greater number of drugs taken, the greater the risk of a drug–drug interaction (DDI) where the taking of one drug aggravates the adverse effects of another. For example, the combination of an anti-inflammatory (such as ibuprofen) that irritates the lining of the stomach with a blood-thinning anticoagulant (such as warfarin) will markedly increase the risk of internal haemorrhage. How often does this happen? In another study, this time of 1500 patients taking again, on average, seven drugs, nearly half had at least one combination that could possibly contribute to a drug–drug interaction. It is scarcely necessary to point out that the figures cited in just these two studies – two-thirds being prescribed an 'inappropriate medication', one half on a therapeutic regime with a potential DDI – might reasonably be described as awesome.

The elderly are vulnerable too to the 'prescribing cascade', an almost bleakly humorous caricature of thoughtless over-treatment, were it not so serious. Consider, for example, a man in his late seventies, fit and active, playing tennis a couple of times a week, 'routinely prescribed', like so many of his age group, a cholesterol-lowering statin. Two months later he consults his doctor with muscular aches and pains for which, in the absence of any obvious explanation, he is prescribed the anti-inflammatory drug ibuprofen. Two months after that, summoned to the surgery for a flu jab, the nurse takes his blood pressure which is found to be raised, warranting treatment with a blood pressure-lowering thiazide diuretic. Another three months passes and he awakes one night with an excruciatingly painful swollen big toe, correctly diagnosed as an acute attack of gout warranting treatment with allopurinol. When he returns as advised a few weeks later to review the situation his doctor checks his blood sugar level, previously normal, but now found to be raised – resulting in a prescription for the anti-diabetic drug metformin. Soon after he develops severe diarrhoea for which, again in the absence of any obvious cause, his doctor prescribes loperamide. At the next consultation he wonders why 'so many things seem to have gone wrong recently' but is reassured that at his age 'These things happen.' And, anyhow, satisfyingly each of his several medical problems have been successfully dealt with.

But were one to scrutinise his several consultations in any detail, it is possible to discern a cascade. The statins cause the muscular aches and pains. These warrant the anti-inflammatories that, in turn, raise the blood pressure, resulting in the prescription of those antihypertensive thiazide diuretics. These increase both the uric acid level and blood sugar – hence the attack of gout and the diabetes. The latter warrants treatment with the anti-diabetic drug metformin, one of whose well-recognised side effects is diarrhoea, hence the loperamide. Thus, the initial prescription for a statin has led to his being drowned (almost literally) by a cascade of six further drugs.

This is, to be sure, a hypothetical case, but almost invariably it is possible to identify in any lengthy list of drugs one or more that have been prescribed to counter the adverse effects of another. Or, as professor of medicine Paula Rachon noted in an article 'Optimising drug treatment for elderly people': 'The prescribing cascade is clearly preventable by carefully considering whether any new medical condition might be the result of an existing treatment.' Quite so.

It is obvious that the more drugs you take, the greater the risk of an adverse reaction from any one of them. But on top of this enhanced risk, crucially, the cumulative effects of polypharmacy – taking more than five different medications – is *on its own account* implicated in causing or exacerbating the sad if only too familiar decline in functioning of later years known depressingly as 'the geriatric syndromes': dementia, recurrent falls, urinary incontinence and poor appetite, resulting in weight loss and under-nutrition. These geriatric syndromes may for most be an inevitable and irreversible consequence of the ageing process itself but, for some at least, reducing the burden of medication may result in an almost Lazarus-like recovery, restoring memory, appetite and mobility and curing their incontinence.

Taken together, the threat posed by drugs to the health of the elderly can be summarised as follows:

- The risk of adverse drug reactions (ADRs) increases from 13 per cent for those taking two drugs to 58 per cent for those taking five, and to 82 per cent for those taking seven or more.
- ADRs have been reported to occur in 35 per cent of those attending hospital as outpatients and 44 per cent of hospital in-patients, and they account for 10 per cent of emergency hospital admissions.
- The risk of a drug–drug interaction is 50 per cent for those taking five or more drugs, rising to 100 per cent for those taking eight or more.

* * *

The remedy for a drug-induced iatrogenic illness could scarcely be simpler and more gratifying – discontinuing the medication. But this requires 'a correct diagnosis', the recognition that the symptom or illness is indeed due to an adverse drug reaction – and that is not necessarily obvious. There is no difficulty when, for example, some otherwise healthy person who has recently started taking a cholesterol-lowering statin develops muscular aches and pains, the temporal proximity of the initiation of treatment to the onset of symptoms being the obvious clue. This can, however, be misleading, as a drug well tolerated for many years may subsequently be responsible for 'delayed' adverse effects. (The experience of professor of cardiology Desmond Julian, whose two potentially fatal beta blocker-induced disturbances of heart rhythm occurred more than a decade after starting treatment, is described in Appendix 2, 'The (Toxic) Cardiac Cocktail'.)

The diagnosis of drug-induced symptoms is a lot trickier when they are more generalised or non-specific – the tiredness, impaired mobility and dizziness that can so readily be misattributed to the progressive decrepitude of passing years ('We put it down to anno domini'), or prompt the standard rebuff from GPs: 'What can you expect at your age?' And it can be very tricky to determine which of the many drugs being taken is the culprit for any specific symptom, or whether, as noted, polypharmacy per se, the cumulative combination of drugs, is responsible for one or other of those geriatric syndromes.

Thus, while the possibility that some new symptom may be due to the side effect of a drug should clearly be considered, tinkering with those drug regimes, stopping one or more drugs to see whether or not this improves matters, may not be sufficient. Rather, the epic scale of polypharmacy-induced iatrogenesis requires a more robust response – a plan or commitment to radically reduce the burden of medicalisation in the elderly. This in turn requires making a crucial distinction between the two main reasons why the drugs were prescribed in the first place. The first category, with which this chapter opened, are those drugs prescribed for the specific purpose of alleviating the distress of specific symptoms: heartburn relieved by acid-suppressant drugs, the misery of the blues by an antidepressant, stiff and painful joints by an anti-inflammatory, and so on. These are known as 'symptomatic' treatments as they address the distress caused by specific *symptoms*. To be sure, each may cause side effects on its own account, warranting its discontinuation, but there is usually some alternative that can be tried in its place. There are no prizes for anticipating the second category of reasons for initiating drug treatment, those 'preventative' medications (antihypertensives, statins, beta blockers, etc.) intended to prevent some misfortune in the future.

Consider, for example, a woman, Mrs Smith, in her late seventies troubled by painful arthritis of the knees and a wheezy chest from chronic obstructive pulmonary disease (COPD). She had a small stroke six years ago following which she was found to have raised blood pressure and blood sugar, leading to a diagnosis of both hypertension and diabetes. More recently she fell and broke her wrist prompting a bone density scan that revealed thinning of the bone (osteoporosis). For all that, she gets by well enough and can scarcely be described as seriously ill. Nonetheless, the current guidelines for treating her several conditions require her to take twelve separate drugs in nineteen separate doses on five separate occasions during the day – including the bone-strengthening drug alendronate once a week. A therapeutic tsunami indeed.

Table 7.1 The burden of polypharmacy in a woman in her seventies with five medical conditions

Conditions	Drug Treatment
Hypertension	hydrochlorothiazide, lisinopril
Diabetes	glyburide, metformin, aspirin and atorvastatin
Osteoarthritis	ibuprofen and paracetamol
Osteoporosis	calcium, vitamin D, alendronate
COPD	bronchodilator

Scrutinising the list of her conditions and medications (see Table 7.1) prompts the immediate observation that just three of the twelve drugs she is taking (paracetamol, the anti-inflammatory ibuprofen and bronchodilator) fall into the first category of 'symptomatic' medicines, alleviating respectively the pain and stiffness of her arthritic joints and the breathlessness due to her wheezy chest. Next it is clearly possible that she might be the unwitting victim of the 'prescribing cascade': anti-inflammatories raise the blood pressure, hence her hypertension, whose treatment with a thiazide diuretic can raise the blood sugar, hence the diabetes and the need for the two different anti-diabetic drugs – metformin and glyburide. Then, for women in her age group, there is no evidence that statins are of value in primary prevention, while the bone-strengthening drug alendronate reduces the likelihood of sustaining a further fracture only modestly. There is thus, as will be seen in the closing chapter, considerable scope for 'rationalising' her drug regime, protecting her against the hazards of polypharmacy by reducing that clearly excessive score of twelve different drugs.

There are millions like her who would similarly benefit from 'rationalisation' of their drug regime, a formidable task that could be made a lot easier by addressing the fundamental issue of why so many of these drugs were prescribed in the first place. This brings us to the central unifying phenomenon that more than anything else accounts for the over-treatment of oldies – and should, were it possible, be announced to the blast of trumpets and clash of cymbals: *Physiological variables rise with age.*

Decade by decade, we see the same strikingly consistent pattern where the 'normal' or average measurement for blood pressure, cholesterol and glucose curves gradually upwards. So, if one wants to track the cholesterol levels in one million people (see Figure 7.1), the mean or average level in their thirties (at 5.5) will by their mid-sixties have risen to 6.5. Now, as described in earlier chapters, the 'experts' over the past thirty years have consistently lowered the threshold or cut-off point for diagnosing hypertension, diabetes and raised cholesterol, with the result

Figure 7.1 The mean (or average) cholesterol level rises with age

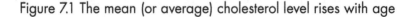
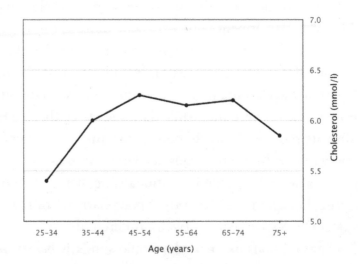

that the vast majority of oldies qualify automatically (because of the rising trend exhibited with age) for drug treatment.

And treated they are. For, as noted in the previous chapter, the readiest way for GPs to maximise their income within the financially incentivised goals of the QOF system is to measure the physiological variables of their older patients. And, hey presto, for three-quarters or more these may be above the threshold warranting treatment to lower them. But are they right to do so? Consider, for example, a man in his early forties, whose cholesterol level of 7.0 is markedly higher than 'normal' for his age group, increasing the subsequent risk of a heart attack that can be reduced, if modestly, by taking statins. But for someone in their seventies, that same cholesterol level has a quite different resonance. It is now only marginally higher than 'average' for his peer group, its contribution to the subsequent risk of a heart attack lower and thus the benefit, if any, of taking statins less. Similar situations apply for blood pressure and glucose, where a systolic pressure of 160, for example, is high for a forty-year-old but 'normal' for a seventy-year-old – and so on. Meanwhile the chance of those in their seventies and beyond experiencing drug-induced side effects from their statins and antihypertensives is much greater than for those in their forties – such that the pay-off, the metric of the benefits and risks of drug treatment, becomes highly equivocal. From all this, one might infer that were doctors to make the necessary adjustments for age, then much over-treatment of the elderly would be avoided – would it not?

Yes, perhaps, but the catch that locks – or coerces – oldies into the straitjacket of over-medication is the blunt response to the oft-asked question 'Do I really need to be taking all these pills?' Namely, 'You would not be here if you stopped taking them.'

The reasoning is as follows. The circulatory disorders of heart disease and stroke are, like all illnesses, profoundly age-determined – the longer you live, the greater the risk of both, as the internal lining of the arteries battered by a lifetime of blood surging through them under pressure becomes progressively harder and narrower. And so, just as the physiological variables of blood pressure and cholesterol rise with age, so the chances of a heart attack or stroke are almost four times greater in seventy-year-olds compared to those in their forties. Now, to be sure, everyone must die of something, but the logic is remorseless. All of us by our seventies have become aware of our mortality, as the prospect of being felled or disabled by some serious medical misfortune becomes ever closer. There is not much that can be done to avoid the 'sniper fire' from any number of types of cancer, but you can to a certain extent control your destiny by reducing (or at least postponing) the risks of those circulatory disorders by taking the pills as recommended by the doctor. It would be absurd not to. There is certainly an even greater incentive to do so than when younger. The bell tolls, and how can one be sure it does not toll for thee?

From the doctor's perspective, the motivations for prescribing blood pressure and cholesterol-lowering medications are rather more complex – leaving aside the financial incentives to do so. He knows (or should know) that these circulatory disorders are an inevitable consequence of ageing and that, for most, the misfortune of having a heart attack or stroke is only marginally, if at all, related to their blood pressure or cholesterol level, which may be within the average range for their age group. But while recognising the very modest benefits of lowering those variables with drug treatment, in prescribing them he is at least 'off the hook' of having to justify to, for example, the relatives of someone recently felled by a stroke, why he has not done so. On the contrary, he has done his best – and ticked the boxes on which his remuneration depends. This is indeed, literally, 'medicine by numbers'.

It is, however, quite contrary to the ethos of 'holistic' care that requires doctors to take into account the wider picture of their patients as individuals, with their own hopes and fears of living out their closing decades to best effect. And that entails protecting them from the hidden hazards of over-medication, whose potentially catastrophic consequences are illustrated by the following cautionary (and tragic) tale:

'Mr O, a bachelor farmer, had never had a serious illness. He enjoyed his beer, tended a small garden, mowed the lawn, drove a vintage pick-up truck and looked after his older brother (aged 92) with early dementia. His first major encounter with the doctor was when he was a robust 80-year-old on no medications. His blood pressure was slightly raised at 150/96 mm of mercury as was his HbA1c at 8.5 per cent. His doctor, following the current guidelines, prescribed an ACE inhibitor and metformin. Both his blood pressure and HbA1c remained stubbornly elevated, so the antihypertensive calcium channel blocker was added along with a second diabetic drug. This had little effect, so the dose of his calcium channel blocker was doubled and he was started on long-acting insulin. The night before his admission to hospital he got up to urinate, fell and broke his hip. When the paramedics arrived, his systolic blood pressure was 80mmHg and his blood sugar showed he was hypoglycaemic. He was given 50 per cent glucose solution with immediate improvement. Around sixteen hours after the fall and fracture, he was taken to the operating room where he had a total hip replacement. While in the recovery room, he was noted to have difficulty using his right hand and was not speaking clearly. Over the next few hours it became clear he had had a stroke. He was started on physical therapy and transferred to a rehabilitation unit where he remained for a further three months, unlikely to ever live independently. Meanwhile, his brother with dementia had to be admitted to a nursing home.

In retrospect, Mr O got into a relentless downward spiral fuelled by interventions based on guidelines to tightly control both his blood sugar and blood pressure – well-recognised targets on which the doctor's performance is judged. His doctor may have been financially rewarded for adhering to those guidelines, but he lost his home and independence.'

Mr O's downward spiral may be a particularly striking instance of the hazards of current medical practice in fetishising the pursuit of 'numerical' goals (the 'optimum' blood pressure and sugar levels) over holistic care, which would have left him to continue enjoying his life 'on no medication'. It is likely to be not untypical: a similar story, or variations on it, accounting for much of the spectacular 75 per cent increase in emergency hospital admissions due to adverse drug reactions. This illuminates with great clarity the curse of those 'thresholds' as they apply to oldies, where a marginally elevated blood pressure and sugar level (normal, as noted, for their age group) initiates an onslaught of drug treatment to bring them in line with those of someone thirty or forty years younger. How did this come about?

Mr O's over-zealous treatment (and that of many like him)

is based on what can best be described as a naive interpretation of the significance of those physiological variables in the elderly and their presumed causative role in the circulatory disorders. The reasoning runs as follows. Heart attacks and strokes are best avoided. Most (three-quarters) occur in those aged seventy and over. Their physiological variables rise with age, so when measured, they are above the threshold to initiate treatment. Ergo, their raised blood pressure and cholesterol levels explain the increased risk of circulatory disorders in the elderly. Thus, it would be negligent of doctors *not* to prescribe blood pressure and cholesterol-lowering medication to the elderly, as they are most likely to benefit from taking them.

The contrary argument would be that rising physiological variables are 'normal' for that age group, while their contributory role in causing circulatory disorders is tenuous, with many heart attacks and strokes a natural and inescapable feature of ageing. Meanwhile (as Mr O's downward spiral illustrates so vividly), there are substantial hazards from the over-zealous pursuit of 'normalising' those physiological variables. For all that, the assumption in favour of prevention as a general principle is so deeply entrenched it would be a brave person who would pass up on the promise that, by taking statins or antihypertensives, they would avoid these serious medical misfortunes in later life – all the more so for those who have already sustained a heart attack or stroke, who will naturally wish to take the necessary precautions to avoid another. The only way out of this bind is to pay attention to the specifics of the benefits and risks of treatment for oldies, while bearing in mind the sensible dictum that their 'drug therapy should be kept to a minimum'. The specifics, as will be seen, are very revealing. We shall consider in turn each of those three physiological variables, and the merits, or otherwise, of medication – starting with a 'raised' cholesterol level.

'Raised' cholesterol

It is almost impossible for those in their seventies and beyond to escape being prescribed a cholesterol-lowering statin for one (or more) reasons:

- *Normal ageing.* Cholesterol levels, as noted, rise with age, thus considerably more than half of those aged seventy and beyond will be above the current 'threshold' for initiating treatment.
- *Cardiac risk score.* The calculation of the cardiac risk (QRisk2) score – the obscure mathematical algorithm predicting the likelihood of a coronary over the next ten years (as considered in Chapter 4) – brings the numbers taking statins to almost 100 per cent. The reasoning is as follows. The longer you live, the greater the risk for coronary; thus incorporation of 'age' into the algorithm means the calculation for most of those aged over seventy will give a score that qualifies them for taking statins.
- *Heart disease.* The incidence of heart disease, as noted, being age-determined, the majority of those experiencing a heart attack will be seventy or over and thus eligible for being prescribed statins as 'secondary prevention' in anticipation of preventing a further episode.
- *Type 2 diabetes.* The chance of being diagnosed with Type 2 diabetes increases with age – and is a further automatic qualification for being prescribed statins.

The evidence of benefit

There would have to be very good reason for the near universal prescription of any powerful drug. But, as a recent review observes:

'Despite their wide-spread use, evidence for the effectiveness of statins in the elderly is unclear. The American Medical Directors Association recommends that they not be routinely prescribed in adults aged seventy years or older based on the lack of an association between high cholesterol levels and outcomes in older adults as well as the potential for an increased risk of adverse events.'

Specifically, the merits of statins for primary prevention in those without a previous history of heart disease (the 'normal ageing' and 'QRisk score' categories above) was investigated in the PROSPER trial, whose findings (as summarised in Chapter 4) were as follows: statins reduce the risk of having a fatal coronary in men by 0.9 per cent (i.e. for 99.1 per cent they make no difference), but have no effect in women and do not prolong life. The situation for those known to have heart disease (the third category above) is slightly better as statins reduce the risk of a further fatal episode by 1.9 per cent. As for diabetes, statins have the two substantial drawbacks of increasing the blood sugar level (thus making it more difficult to control), while not significantly reducing their increased risk of cardiovascular disease.

Harm

The evidence for and testimony to the adverse effects of statins, particularly in oldies, are by now familiar enough, significantly compromising the quality of life in numerous ways from causing crippling muscular aches and pains to inducing a dementia-type syndrome.

Verdict

There is no justification for the current near-universal prescribing of statins for oldies. Their very modest benefits in primary prevention – for men only – and in secondary prevention for those with heart disease must be offset against the likelihood of adverse effects in those taking them.

Hypertension

There is no disputing the imperative of treating raised blood pressure, whose causative role in stroke is much greater than cholesterol for heart disease. The imagery of blood surging through the arteries under pressure bursting a blood vessel and haemorrhaging into the brain could scarcely be more persuasive. And, as considered in Chapter 2, the demonstration of the effectiveness of treatment ranks among the most significant achievements of modern medicine. The same consideration should apply in even greater measure to the elderly – the steep rise of the systolic pressure with age to levels of 170 mmHg or more is paralleled by a similar steep rise in the incidence of stroke. And yet, till the 1990s, doctors were almost surprisingly reluctant to initiate treatment. The rise of the systolic pressure, the argument went, was a normal physiological response to the progressive hardening and narrowing of the arteries requiring a higher pressure to perfuse the brain that, compromised by treatment to lower it, would predispose to falls and other medical misfortunes. Hence the admittedly rather arbitrary 'rule of thumb' whereby a 'normal' systolic blood pressure for the elderly was defined as 100 plus the patient's age – which for someone aged eighty is a seemingly alarming 180. In the early 1990s this rule of thumb was rudely overturned.

The evidence of benefit

The suspicion that those high systolic blood pressures might be dangerous prompted the Systolic Hypertension in the Elderly Program (SHEP), involving 5000 people with an average age of seventy-two. Over a period of five years, the reduction with drug treatment of a systolic pressure of 170 down to just over 140 was found to reduce the number of strokes by 36 per cent and heart attacks by 27 per cent. The previously relaxed attitude to those raised systolic pressures was no longer tenable or, as the organisers of the trial observed: 'There is considerable potential for decreasing morbidity and mortality by effective sustained drug treatment.'

Predictably, the absolute benefit for any individual was much less than these very impressive figures imply: just 2.2 per cent benefiting from a reduced risk of stroke (the difference between the 4.0 per cent on treatment who suffered a stroke, compared to the 6.2 per cent on placebo). Still, there are few more desirable goals of preventive treatment, and it would seem more than worthwhile to treat 2400 people for five years if this means preventing fifty of them experiencing a stroke. It thus almost verges on the negligent not to treat oldies down to the current threshold of 150/80. Still, caution is necessary, for despite the fifty fewer strokes occurring in the 2400 on treatment in the SHEP trial, there was no improvement in overall survival, which is surprising given that strokes are not infrequently fatal. The reason for this anomalous finding becomes apparent when we turn to consider the harms.

Harms

The corollary of those millions of people taking antihypertensives in anticipation of reducing their risk of stroke is that adverse effects are common, so it is only sensible to be aware of the many problems they can cause. The more serious (summarised earlier in Table 3 in Chapter 2) are the depletion of the body's salts (sodium and potassium) with thiazide diuretics and the slowing of the heart with beta blockers, both of which can predispose to serious disturbances of heart rhythm. The further substantial problem with the mass prescribing of antihypertensives is that, for oldies in particular, 'Too much of a good thing can be bad for you'. While it might be desirable to reduce the systolic pressure to 150 mmHg, much lower than this and one starts to run into trouble, as the pressure may be insufficient to propel blood from the heart through the narrowed arteries to the brain. This may manifest itself in two forms.

First, those whose systolic pressure is running at around 120 may experience variously fatigue, weakness, unsteadiness and confusion, all of which may improve dramatically upon reducing the dose or discontinuing the medication.

'My doctor prescribed amlodipine for my raised blood pressure, 5mg at first and increased to 10mg after a month. I then began feeling progressively more and more lethargic until I couldn't even be bothered to turn on the television while I passed my days on the sofa. My blood pressure had indeed gone down (sometimes to less than 100) but this wasn't living! So, I stopped the medication and immediately felt 100 per cent better. Clearly, my BP was too low for me to function properly. I have since lost a little weight and increased my exercise so that it is now around 130/85 on no treatment – so all is well and good.'

The second manifestation of over-treatment is the sudden precipitous fall in blood pressure on standing known as postural hypotension. To clarify, the maintenance of a 'constant' blood pressure is a most complex process, involving a dozen different homeostatic mechanisms that ensure we do not, for example, keel over when rising from the horizontal position in a warm bed at night to the vertical as we head for the bathroom. These homeostatic mechanisms become less efficient with age and are compounded by taking antihypertensives. Hence, as geriatrician Dr John Morley observes, 'Postural hypotension is an extremely common problem in older persons' – with predictably serious consequences:

'My brother, aged 83, has been taking tablets for high blood pressure for some time and has been having episodes of dizziness and balance problems. A few weeks ago, he went to answer his front door bell and just dropped like a stone, hitting his face on the threshold of the door, resulting in various fractures of his cheekbones and a split lip. He was in hospital for a couple of weeks and then two weeks after returning home a similar thing happened but this time he at least managed to sit down before falling.'

Falls, it is scarcely necessary to point out, are bad news, but particularly so when they result in the most serious of fractures, that of the neck of the femur, requiring a major hip replacement operation. This is, of course, a very successful procedure, but for older patients confined to bed, with the attendant risks of blood clots and pneumonia and post-operative complications, the prognosis can be gloomy, resulting for one in ten in a fatal outcome. Here lies the probable explanation for the seemingly anomalous finding, alluded to above, that the SHEP trial did not improve overall survival, the benefit of preventing strokes being offset by the potentially lethal fractures that occur as a result of treatment-induced falls.

Verdict

The rise of the systolic pressure with age is not necessarily benign. Still, caution is necessary in seeking to reduce it to that threshold of 150, paying special attention to the many potential adverse effects of medication and the insidious symptoms of fatigue and unsteadiness that may be due to over-treatment. The substantial dangers of postural hypotension can be avoided by ensuring the blood pressure is measured not only when sitting but also when standing, and preferably after mild exertion, to detect its precipitous drop.

Diabetes

The number of people diagnosed with diabetes increases three-fold between the ages of forty-five and sixty-five, with a prevalence of 15 per cent – rather less than those deemed to have a 'raised' cholesterol or hypertension, but still substantial. For some, no doubt, the diagnosis will be made following investigation of the characteristic symptoms of excess thirst and urination. But most, otherwise fit and well, will be informed of their condition follow-ing a blood test which shows HbA1c to be above the diagnostic threshold of 6.5 (or a blood sugar of 7.0 mmol/L). The controversy surrounding the diagnosis, benefits and harms of treatment has already been discussed in some detail in Chapter 5. It is revisited here with special consideration as to how it applies to oldies.

The evidence of benefit

The necessity for treatment is self-evident in those with symptomatic diabetes, who will feel much better once the several consequences of their raised blood sugar are brought under control. The overweight, being particularly prone to the condition, will be rewarded in their efforts to lose those excess pounds (or stones) by adopting a low carbohydrate diet. The main goal of treatment is to prevent two sets of serious complications – the macrovascular (heart disease, stroke and peripheral vascular disease), and the microvascular (impaired functioning of the kidneys, eyes and nerves). Regrettably these are not, as originally anticipated, completely preventable by the pursuit of 'tight' control, seeking to reduce that HbA1c to 7.5 or less. The rising prevalence of diabetes with age is closely related to the tendency to put on weight as the years tick by from eating (and drinking) more and exercising less, a process reversible by losing weight and cutting back on carbohydrates in favour of meat and dairy products. The prevailing dietary orthodoxy favouring a high carbohydrate diet (as discussed in some detail in Chapter 5) turns this common-sense advice on its head, making it more difficult to lose weight and pushing up the blood sugar, thus increasing the need for drug therapy – an iatrogenic catastrophe indeed.

The second major harm, as with hypertension, comes with over-treatment in pursuit of the target goal of an HbA1c of 7.5 – predisposing the individual to hypoglycaemia (or excessively low blood sugar), the resulting confusion or coma warranting medical intervention or hospital admission to correct it. And, as with hypertension, oldies are particularly vulnerable because of those age-impaired homeostatic mechanisms for maintaining their blood sugar level. So, from 2004 onwards, with GPs now financially incentivised to hit their target thresholds, the number of people requiring treatment for their drug-induced hypoglycaemia has soared: an additional 4000 hospital admissions a year, up from 7868 to 11,756 in 2010 – three-quarters of whom were aged sixty or over. The low blood sugar or hypoglycaemia itself may be readily correctable with an intravenous infusion of a glucose solution but the preceding mental confusion predisposes to serious injuries sustained in road traffic accidents and falls – with the same unfortunate consequences as for postural hypotension.

Verdict

Those alarming figures of the increase in hospital admissions for drug-induced hypoglycaemic confusion or coma are the most conspicuous, and medically measurable, indication of inappropriate or over-treatment of those three physiological variables. They would be avoided – for those who are unable to achieve remission from their diabetes by dietary means – by revising those HbA1c targets upwards from 7.5 to 8–9.

The oldest oldies

The vulnerability of the oldest oldies (those aged eighty-five and over) to the harms of polypharmacy and over-treatment is, for obvious reasons, greater still, though the arguments in favour of reducing the burden of medication are much simpler. From one's eighth decade, the continuous rise of those physiological variables with age plateaus and the association of raised blood pressure and cholesterol with strokes and heart attacks becomes more tenuous still. Instead, now, the *lower* they are, the greater the risk of dying; specifically, in those aged eighty and over, 'Low cholesterol is associated with the highest mortality rate' and 'A low systolic blood pressure is associated with increased mortality'. So there can be no grounds for prescribing medicines to lower them still further. Thus, logically, such prescriptions should be discontinued, not least because stopping statins was found in one study to 'improve the quality of life and reduce the need for medication', while in another the finding that a low systolic pressure in those taking two or more antihypertensive medications doubled the risk of dying prompted the recommendation that 'drug therapy should be reduced'.

Logical perhaps, but doctors and patients alike may be reluctant to reduce or stop their medication, not least because a substantial proportion may have already sustained a heart attack or stroke and will thus be anxious to prevent another. They may indeed view taking antihypertensives and statins as almost a lucky charm, protecting them against, or at least postponing, such an eventuality. The recent, unexpected and dramatic decline in life expectancy alluded to above might persuade them otherwise. The seeming paradox that a systematic approach to discontinuing medicines in this age group may both improve the quality and prolong the lives of many will be considered in the closing chapter, where we examine the practicalities of the advice 'Don't keep taking the pills'.

Chapter 8

Rolling Back the Harms

There are many reasons why it may be desirable to withdraw a medicine: lack of efficacy, actual or potential adverse drug reactions, non-adherence, resolution of the condition, development of a contra indication, introduction of an interacting drug, to name a few.

David Alldred, 'Deprescribing: A brave new word?', *International Journal of Pharmacy Prescribing* (2014)

Polypharmacy may, by common consent, be an aberration but for all the persuasive evidence of, for many, the minuscule benefits and potentially substantial harms, it remains as deeply entrenched as ever. And will remain so until the false premises of the 'population approach' are revoked and GPs are no longer financially incentivised to implement it. So, what is to be done?

The guiding principle for 'rolling back the harms' was proposed more than fifteen years ago by the then editor of the *British Medical Journal*, Dr Richard Smith, in a prescient editorial, 'Too much medicine? Almost certainly'. The public, 'ordinary people', he suggested, must 'increasingly take charge ... weighing the costs and benefits of the medicalisation of their lives'. Then, 'Armed with better information about the natural course of common conditions, they can more judiciously assess the real value of medicine's never-ending regimen of tests and treatments.'

This closing chapter will explore how that principle can be turned into reality. For while it is only sensible to defer to the experience and expertise of doctors, they clearly need to be encouraged to be rather more self-critical about their profligate prescribing. There are indeed 'many reasons' why (as the introductory quote has it) 'It may be desirable to withdraw a medicine', so it is necessary to appreciate first why doctors might be reluctant to do so. Dr Ian Scott of the University of Queensland has identified four barriers to 'deprescribing' – defined as 'systematically identifying and tapering, reducing or stopping medications that are not indicated or have potential to cause adverse effects'. The main barrier, not surprisingly, is 'lack of awareness of the scale and impact of inappropriate polypharmacy'. The defining feature of the current epidemic of iatrogenic illness is that the symptoms of fatigue, impaired mobility and general decrepitude can so readily be misattributed, by both patients and doctors, to 'getting on'.

Then, deprescribing may be perceived as a risky affair. This obviously applies particularly to drugs intended to prevent some misfortune in the future. Here doctors are, not unreasonably, fearful of criticism from colleagues or relatives if their discontinuing a drug is followed by some untoward event – or, as one GP put it: 'The reason we don't like stopping medication is, uh, coincidentally that the patient might die and we will be blamed for it.' Then they might, again reasonably, be reluctant to ignore or contradict the advice of a specialist – 'So, they have seen the cardiologist and been started on a statin. You then feel nervous about stopping it even if it seems to be the right thing to do.' Similar considerations apply when the GP initiates treatment on his own account in line with 'current guidelines' mandated by expert committees who might be presumed (not necessarily correctly) to base their recommendations on a dispassionate evaluation of the relevant scientific evidence. And finally, doctors may simply feel they do not have the time in the busy routine of everyday general practice to question whether one drug or another is still necessary, or to search back through a patient's records to find out why it was prescribed in the first place. It is certainly much simpler just to sign off the pile of repeat prescriptions sitting on the desk.

For all that, when 90 per cent of those GPs in the straw poll mentioned in the Introduction acknowledge that they are prescribing 'too many pills', they are clearly open to the proposal that they prescribe fewer – and if prompted to do so at their patients' request, then these 'barriers' to deprescribing are more readily surmountable. This is the preferred option: for while several of those cited in previous chapters have resorted to unilateral action, discontinuing their medication in defiance of their doctor's advice, a collaborative approach is much more desirable for any number of common-sense reasons.

Most doctors, one hopes, would welcome the opportunity to

improve the quality of their patients' lives, perhaps markedly so, by reviewing and rationalising their drug regime. Still, no doubt this can be a tricky situation and some 'prior research' is essential. This, gratefully, is easily done, as the central argument surrounding each of the five pillars of polypharmacy examined in this book is encapsulated in a single article that can be downloaded from the internet or obtained from the local library (see Table 8.1). They have, inevitably, the usual quota of technical jargon, but the gist, interpreted within the context of the relevant chapter, is clear enough.

Table 8.1 The five pillars of polypharmacy: The verdict

Hypertension	'This review found that compared with a placebo, treatment with an antihypertensive drug did not reduce any outcome including total mortality, total cardiovascular events, coronary heart disease or stroke.' Professor Stephen Martin, 'Mild hypertension in people at low risk', *British Medical Journal*, 349 (2014): g5432
'Raised' cholesterol	'Statin therapy in those at low risk does not reduce overall mortality or serious illness with an increased risk of causing side effects that range from minor and reversible to serious and irreversible.' Dr John D. Abramson, 'Should people at low risk of cardiovascular disease take a statin?', *British Medical Journal*, 347 (2013): f6123
Diabetes	'A low carbohydrate diet resulted in substantial weight loss in all patients and brought about normalisation of blood glucose. Seven patients were able to come off medication.' Dr David Unwin, 'The low carbohydrate diet to achieve weight loss and improve HbA1c Type 2 diabetes', *Practical Diabetes*, vol. 31 (2014), pp. 1–4

Osteoporosis	'[Drug treatment] can achieve at best a marginal reduction in hip fractures at the cost of serious medical adverse events and forgone opportunities to have a great impact on the health of older people.' Teppo Jarvinen, *British Medical Journal*, 350 (2015): h2088
Cardiac cocktail	'It is important to challenge the assumption that the efficacy and safety of drugs given in the relatively short term remain the same over the long term.' Professor Desmond Julian, 'Long-term use of cardiovascular drugs', *Journal of the American College of Cardiology*, 66 (2015), pp. 1273–85

The only other essential resource is 'A Practical Guide to Stopping Medicines', which despite the disclaimer that 'some content may no longer be current' (having been published in 2010) is still the most readily accessible summary of the rationale for deprescribing.

So, 'Armed with this better information', much more definitive than when the editor of the *BMJ* wrote his challenging editorial fifteen years ago – how do ordinary people 'judiciously assess the real value of medicine's never-ending regimen of tests and treatments'?

There are two distinct scenarios here. The first is the person who may have been taking one (or more) of the five 'pillars' of polypharmacy for several years and may reasonably wonder whether it is necessary to continue doing so indefinitely. The second concerns those afflicted with several medical conditions and taking half a dozen or more different drugs where, it is argued by some, deprescribing may need to be much more radical.

First scenario

*It makes no sense at all to take a drug intended
to prevent some medical condition in the future
if it is causing you problems now.*

Dr Andrew Herxheimer, 'Golden Rules of
Drug Therapy'

Times change, and while in the past doctors may have defensively dismissed concerns about the burdens of medication, most now would respond sympathetically to a patient's complaint that she is 'taking too many pills'. Still, they may need to be encouraged to reconsider whether the drugs they routinely prescribe may be discontinued by one of 'several triggers' – the first being that they might be responsible for 'hidden' side effects masquerading as the tribulations of ageing. This 'premature ageing' can be quite subtle, only becoming apparent with the gratifying rebound in general health and robustness when the medication is discontinued.

The further trigger has to be any symptom that remains unexplained despite referral to a specialist whose thorough investigations have failed to identify what is amiss. Indeed, the spectrum of possible adverse effects is so protean that any puzzling symptom must be presumed to be drug-induced – unless proved otherwise.

The third trigger for discontinuing medication – vividly illustrated in the epilogue to Chapter 5, 'A master class in deprescribing' – is where a change in lifestyle (losing weight, abstemious drinking and taking more exercise) 'normalises' those physiological variables such that within a few months Mr Y was able to stop all his medication. There is no reason why the legions of those ranging from the 'pleasantly plump' to the seriously overweight might not benefit in a similar way.

We turn now to highlight some further considerations in promoting the cause of deprescribing – with reference to Table 8.1 – for three of those pillars of polypharmacy. The remaining two, osteoporosis and the cardiac cocktail, are considered in some detail in the two appendices.

Mild hypertension

The scope for deprescribing here is prodigious. Two-thirds of those taking blood pressure-lowering drugs have 'mild' hypertension (140–159/90–99), for which we now know those drugs confer no benefit, whether in reducing the subsequent risk of heart attack or stroke or prolonging life. The corollary of this is that those whose blood pressure is below these measurements may be being 'over-treated', particularly if they are experiencing fatigue or dizziness. The further relevant points to be considered are:

- Blood pressure is the most 'variable' of the physiological variables, a fact readily apparent from its tendency to fluctuate markedly when measured repeatedly over a period of five to ten minutes. Hence the recommendation that all those diagnosed with hypertension should purchase a home monitoring device as the simplest and most reliable way of establishing the 'true' blood pressure.
- For one in ten (or more) of those diagnosed with hypertension the blood pressure will subsequently fall back within the normal range without the need for medication.

- The two most widely prescribed antihypertensive drugs associated with adverse effects are the thiazide diuretics such as bendrofluazide (diabetes and gout) and the beta blockers (fatigue and disturbances of heart rhythm). These should, if possible, be avoided.

'Raised' cholesterol

Here the scope for deprescribing parallels that for mild hypertension, where two-thirds of those taking statins are doing so for 'primary' prevention; in whom, as Dr John Abramson reports, 'they neither prevent serious illness nor prolong survival'. This verdict is, to be sure, disputed, so the decision as to whether to continue taking statins indefinitely then depends on whose interpretation of the evidence is felt to be the more credible. Some may be persuaded by the verdict of the major review of the twenty-seven drug company-sponsored clinical trials that statins are wonder drugs of value for everyone (young and old, male and female, those at low and high risk, etc.) while also being 'remarkably safe'. Others, noting the minuscule absolute benefit as revealed by the Numbers Needed to Treat (see Figure 4.4), may take a contrary view. They might also be sceptical of the 'coronary risk score', on the basis of whose obscure mathematical calculations 85 per cent of those aged sixty-five and over are at 'high risk' and are deemed eligible to take statins. The score, as recently noted, overestimates the true risk of a coronary by between five- and six-fold.

Diabetes

There is less scope for deprescribing in those with Type 2 diabetes but, as noted, it is for many a reversible condition with appropriate changes in diet and losing weight, thus minimising, or indeed obviating, the need for medication.

The practicalities of deprescribing in this first scenario are fairly straightforward. It seems only sensible that those taking statins should periodically take a drug-free holiday for a month or two to see whether this improves any 'hidden' symptoms of decrepitude, followed by an informed discussion as to whether they should be restarted. And it is only sensible too to monitor the effects of tapering antihypertensive and diabetic drugs in those who have made 'appropriate lifestyle changes' and whose blood pressure or sugar level is at or below the recommended threshold. This may allow for the dosage to be reduced or for the drugs to be discontinued altogether.

Second scenario

> *Polypharmacy is the disease and thus the specific treatment is simple: stopping as many medications as possible. Deprescribing is the cure.*
>
> Doron Garfinkel, *Therapeutic Advances in Drug Safety*

The options for deprescribing in the second scenario – for those taking half a dozen or more drugs for several medical conditions – are inevitably more complex and time-consuming, though the potential benefits are greater still. Here the practicalities are best illustrated by reference to 79-year-old Mrs Smith, encountered in the previous chapter, who, as may be recalled, following a stroke six years ago and more recently a fractured wrist, is now taking twelve different drugs in nineteen separate doses five times a day. These are intended to mitigate variously the discomforts of her painful arthritic knees and wheezy chest, to control her hypertension and diabetes and prevent a further fracture (see Table 7.1). For all that, she is well enough, though not as active as she would wish, troubled at times by dizziness and sleeping poorly. Her polypharmacy increases the risk of subsequently developing one or other of those 'geriatric syndromes' (dementia, recurrent falls, undernourishment and urinary incontinence) or requiring emergency hospital admission either for an adverse effect of one or other of her medications or as a consequence of over-treatment resulting in low blood pressure or blood sugar level. There is, as noted, the clear possibility that she may be an unwitting victim of the prescribing cascade: the anti-inflammatory she is taking for her arthritis raising her blood pressure, whose treatment with a thiazide diuretic increases her blood sugar and thus the need for the two anti-diabetic drugs, metformin and glyburide. How to proceed?

Though fully recovered from her stroke, Mrs Smith, and certainly her doctor, will wish, for obvious reasons, to continue with her antihypertensive drugs. Still, her complaint of dizziness suggests she may be being over-treated and, if so, her doctor might consider discontinuing the thiazide diuretic. This would have the further advantage, as thiazides raise the blood sugar, of allowing her to reduce the dose of her anti-diabetic drugs or, better still, when combined with a low carbohydrate diet, permit her to stop the glyburide. She might also take a statin holiday to see whether this allows her to be more active – it may be contributing to the aches and pains associated with her arthritis – and improves her insomnia. As for the bone-strengthening

alendronate, its benefits, despite the osteoporosis and wrist fracture, are (as discussed in Appendix 1) modest, and the prevailing
view would be that it can be discontinued after five years. She
should continue with the aspirin and the three 'symptomatic'
drugs: the paracetamol, the anti-inflammatory ibuprofen for her
arthritis and the inhaler for her wheezy chest.

The merits of rationalising her drug regime in this way should
be self-evident, with the prospect of markedly improving her life
both now and in the future. When the previously mentioned
Dr Ian Scott undertook a similar exercise in fifty patients who,
like Mrs Smith, were taking eight or more regularly prescribed
drugs, he was able to discontinue one-third – most commonly
statins, antihypertensives, acid suppressants and anti-diabetic
drugs. Over the following four months, just over 1 per cent of
those discontinued drugs had to be restarted.

The scope for improving the quality of life for many by reducing
the burden of their polypharmacy is thus considerable but –
beyond the findings of Dr Doron Garfinkel's study of how
deprescribing prolonged the lives of nursing home residents,
mentioned in the previous chapter – there is as yet little 'hard'
evidence that it is as beneficial as might be anticipated. This
brings us back to the question posed in the opening chapter, as
to whether polypharmacy might be a contributory factor to the
recently noted decline in life expectancy in Britain and elsewhere.

We return first to the driving force behind escalating polypharmacy, the very influential 'population theory' proposed by
epidemiologist Geoffrey Rose back in the 1980s – the supposition that the 'population was sick'. Then we noted at the close
of Chapter 6 how the immensely costly QOF system had inadvertently tested the claim that 'population approach'-induced

polypharmacy would 'save' an estimated 30,000 lives a year. On the contrary, it had zero effect in improving survival. The converse of the failure of polypharmacy to do good is almost certainly that it will be harmful. It can, as noted, be fatal, killing people before their time in three distinct ways: first, by being responsible for the sharp rise in emergency hospital admissions for adverse drug reactions (with a 10 per cent fatality rate); next, by inducing the state of decrepitude of the 'geriatric syndromes'; and, finally, through over-treatment predisposing to potentially fatal falls and similar misfortunes.

There is, of course, no way of knowing how many lives polypharmacy may have cost. For, as observed, shamefully there is no systematic method for collecting the relevant data. But sooner or later those drug-induced fatalities will have an influence on life expectancy, and indeed within a few years of the institutionalisation of mass medication (via the QOF), it stalled and then went into reverse. And by how much? There is a memorable, if disturbing symmetry in the relevant statistics where, far from polypharmacy 'saving' 30,000 lives annually, there were an estimated 30,000 more deaths in 2015 compared to the previous year. The same phenomenon of declining life expectancy is apparent in other Western European countries (France, Germany, Italy and the United States), all of which have witnessed the same massive upswing in polypharmacy. Thus, while there is, to be sure, no definitive proof as yet that polypharmacy is the culprit, the circumstantial evidence is strongly persuasive. There is, however, one simple way by which this issue can be clarified – and that is for doctors to reduce markedly the number of drugs prescribed in the ways outlined above and observe whether that decline in life expectancy is reversed. Time will tell.

Appendix 1

Fractured Follies

'I don't have Monday morning blues – I get them on Tuesdays instead. That's when I have to take my "bone pill": alendronate, a commonly prescribed drug for osteoporosis. I religiously follow the instructions: to swallow the tablet with a large glass of tap water, stay fully upright afterwards and neither eat nor drink for at least thirty minutes. So, no early morning cup of tea, no breakfast and no going back to bed either. It may sound feeble but I have come to dread this early morning ritual. I tell myself I am lucky, thanks to sophisticated scanning techniques my osteoporosis was diagnosed early (at 55) while the development of drugs such as alendronate (called bisphosphonates) means, so the specialists tell me, that my weakened bones can be rebuilt and any future risk of painful and disabling fractures reduced. But two years after starting this treatment, I am still ambivalent about it. Every week I wonder whether or not to take my tablets. And, judging by the agonised discussions on internet forums, there are thousands of women in my position who feel the same.'

Cherrill Hicks, Daily Telegraph, 2010

'For several years now I have been taking a bisphosphonate for bone strengthening. This was on the advice of my GP who told me that, without it, it would be "downhill all the way". A few weeks ago, I made an appointment at the surgery to see if there was anything more effective, after all medicines are always being improved on. This time I learnt there was absolutely no need to take any bone-strengthening medicine. A good diet of dairy products, plenty of sunlight and walking was good enough. She promptly cancelled my prescription.'

Mrs B. S., 2011

We might all wish to grow old gracefully, but the combined hazards of the increasing predisposition with passing years to falling over and thinning of the bones means that some time or another one in two women and one in four men will sustain a traumatic fracture. The commonest, by far, are compression fractures of the vertebrae – an estimated 120,000 a year in Britain – whether spontaneous, due simply to the downward force of gravity on the spinal column, or precipitated by some seemingly trivial event such as sneezing or a sudden change in position. Next come the 'Colles' fractures of the wrist – 46,000 a year from falling on an outstretched hand or slipping on an icy or leaf-strewn pavement. Then the most grievous of all, the fractured hip, 25,000 a year, warranting the immensely successful operation of a hip replacement that nonetheless for the frail may be a terminal event, the 'final straw' that brings their lives to a close.

Taken together that adds up to a substantial burden of pain, suffering, disability and death, one that is scarcely truly preventable but may in some instances be avoidable by means of bone-strengthening drugs that counter the inevitable thinning of the bones with age known as osteoporosis. The simplest and most effective treatment is Hormone Replacement Therapy (HRT). The structural integrity of bone, as all know, is strikingly compromised by the fall in oestrogen levels associated with the menopause – warranting a brief diversionary clarification.

Bones are an engineering marvel, light, flexible and strong, constantly remodelling themselves as they grow in size in response to the changing forces imposed upon them. Thus, the humerus of the upper arm, at birth a mere four inches of bendy cartilage linking the shoulder to the elbow joint, over the years to adulthood increases four-fold in length to become a powerful mobile lever capable of performing a vast range of different movements.

At any moment during those early years, scrutinising a cross-section of bone through a magnifying glass – were that possible – would reveal (almost literally) a hive of activity. For just as bees are skilful masons busily fabricating the cells of their honeycombs from the waxy secretions of their bodies, so too armies of minuscule cells are constantly remodelling the internal structure of the bones.

First, millions of demolition workers (the osteoclasts) clear the site, boring holes through the bone, liquidising it with their potent acidic secretions, creating long tunnels that coalesce into cavities. In their wake come waves of builders (or osteoblasts), filling those cavities with a hard mixture of calcium and phosphate. This continuous cycle of bone remodelling takes place in a coordinated fashion known as 'coupling', where each army of 'clasts' and 'blasts', it must be presumed, somehow knows what the other is doing.

Their activities in turn are guided and influenced by a higher power outside themselves, the ever-changing and increasing mechanical loads imposed on the humerus as its possessor matures through childhood into adolescence. Thus, year by year, the 'form' or internal structure of bone is being continually realigned with the stresses involved in normal skeletal function.

Like painting the Forth Bridge, this remodelling by the armies of clasts and blasts continues throughout adult life. But come the menopause, the falling level of oestrogen, for reasons that are not at all clear, accelerates the process, and the frequency of those cycles of remodelling become ever more frenetic. The clasts (as it were) gain the upper hand, removing more bone than the blasts can replace; the internal architecture of bone with its supporting struts (or trabeculae) becomes thinner and the bone more porous (hence osteoporosis). There is no escaping this biologically determined post-menopausal thinning of the bone. For some women it may be particularly severe, as summarised in this composite description of a woman in her early sixties:

'She first notices weakness and a dull ache in the lower part of the back that is aggravated following a slight jar or fall, resulting in often agonising pains that may persist for weeks. As the condition progresses, spinal deformity develops, usually a rounded kyphosis – the dowager's hump – of the upper thorax with considerable limitations of spinal movements due to muscle spasm. The most striking X-ray change is a uniform thinning of the affected bones, chiefly of the spine and pelvis. In the lower spine, the vertebrae become concave and wedge-shaped, followed by actual collapse of the vertebral body itself.'

The advent of HRT in the 1960s promised to halt this remorseless process in its tracks. And indeed it did, as first demonstrated in a decade-long study published in 1979 comparing the outcome in two groups of eighty-four women allocated to receive either a placebo pill or a combination of oestrogen and progesterone. After ten years, the bone mass of those taking the placebo had declined on average by 15 per cent, some seven of them sustaining a major fracture. Those taking HRT, by contrast, had 'minimal' bone loss, without a single fracture. 'When oestrogens are administered within three years of the menopause,' observed Professor Leila Nachtigall of the New York University Medical Centre, 'osteoporosis can actually be reversed.'

This finding has been replicated many times and is a major factor in the common perception of HRT as virtually a panacea against the physical effects of ageing – leaving aside its indubitable merits in countering the distressing subjective symptoms of hot flushes, insomnia, low mood, muscular aches and pains, vaginal dryness and so on. There were, it seemed, only two drawbacks. First, not all women wished to take HRT, and certainly not indefinitely – for once it is discontinued, its protective effect in maintaining bone mass is lost. Then, if obviously, it is scarcely an option for men.

Still, HRT undoubtedly protects against osteoporosis – and would continue to do so, were it not for its dramatic fall from grace in 2002 with the surprising verdict of the Women's Health Initiative study (involving almost 20,000 women) that, on balance, it did 'more harm than good'. That possibility of harm was, for any individual, small, but while 5 out of 10,000 women taking HRT for a year might expect to be protected against sustaining a fractured hip, this was at the cost of seven more heart attacks, eight more strokes and eight more cases of invasive breast cancer. This verdict, it has subsequently been claimed, exaggerated the scale of those harms, but at the time it effectively subverted any prospect that HRT might be a realistic long-term solution. But it had certainly raised expectations, preparing the way, as it were, for the next pharmacological assault on osteoporosis-related fractures that the drug company Merck (who else?) had been planning for the previous two decades.

Back in 1982 Merck secured the worldwide licence to develop alendronate, one of a class of chemicals known as the bisphosphonates that possess the unique and remarkable property of selectively blocking the action of the armies of bone-munching osteoclasts, thus inhibiting the intensive cycles of remodelling that, as considered above, become ever more frenetic following the menopause.

Merck at the time (as may be recalled from Chapter 4) was preparing to launch the first cholesterol-lowering statin, Mevacor, with a marketing strategy aimed, as its former chairman Henry Gadsden had put it, at 'selling to everyone'. The spectacular rise of statins would, in turn, provide a model for the promotion of alendronate, both for 'primary prevention' of fractures in those without any overt symptoms of osteoporosis and 'secondary prevention' for those who had already sustained a fracture in the expectation of avoiding another one. The practicalities were, however, much more complex. It was straightforward to promote statins by encouraging everyone to 'know their number' (i.e. their cholesterol level) by visiting their doctor for the simple blood test that would indicate if they were above the 'threshold' for initiating treatment. But the comparable screening method for osteoporosis requires rather a sophisticated and costly device, the Dexa-scanner (or Dual-energy X-ray absorptiometry) that utilises two X-ray beams of different energies to determine the Bone Mineral Density that is expressed as a single number or 'T-score'. And where to draw the line between a 'normal' and an 'abnormal' T-score?

In 1992, a group of osteoporosis experts, chaired by Professor John Kanis of the University of Sheffield, convened in Rome to deliberate this question under the auspices of the World Health Organisation. The benchmark for 'normal', they resolved, should be the T-score measurement typical of a 'healthy young adult woman'. And the abnormal?

'Ultimately it was just a matter of, "Well ... the line has to be drawn somewhere",' recalls Professor Anna Tosteson of Dartmouth Medical School. 'It was very hot in the room, people were in shirt sleeves and, you know, it was time to move on, as it were. I can't quite frankly remember who it was who stood up and drew a line through the graph depicting diminishing bone density and decreed: every woman on one side of this line has osteoporosis.'

The report of the meeting, subsequently published as 'Assessment of factor risk and its application to screening for osteoporosis', conceded that this cut-off point was 'somewhat arbitrary', but confirmed that a T-score of –2.5 or less should be diagnostic of osteoporosis (a measurement of 2.5 standard deviations below 'normal'). Those in whom the score fell in the range of –1 to –2.5 had the precursor state of 'osteopenia' – literally 'poverty of bone'.

This reduction of osteoporosis to a single numerical score certainly simplified matters, though as will be seen it did not necessarily reflect the realities of the relationship between the density of bone and the subsequent risk of fracture. Thus, the fittest of footballers with a normal T-score may break a bone on colliding with one of the opposing team, while a frail granny with a low T-score may never do so – unless she has the misfortune to slip on an icy pavement. The point readily overlooked (or obscured) is that when it comes to predicting the risk of fracture, bone density is considerably less than half the story – and thus the benefit of a drug that inhibits those bone-munching osteoclasts is likely to be modest.

Still, the World Health Organisation's numerical definition would be widely endorsed, and – being readily comprehensible to doctors and public alike – would provide the rationale for a major screening programme where all over a certain age would be encouraged to have a Dexa-scan. Then, those in whom the T-score fell below the 'somewhat arbitrary' WHO definition of osteoporosis became candidates for 'bone-strengthening' drugs. The parallel with the strategy for promoting cholesterol-lowering statins is obvious enough, with a potential market on a similarly epic scale. In the United States alone, 10 million people, it was estimated, had a T-score of –2.5 or less and a further 34 million fell within the osteopenia category. Thus, the osteoporosis experts meeting in Rome, unwittingly or not, had done Merck a massive favour with their authoritative delineation of the potential market for alendronate. All Merck had to do was demonstrate that it did indeed reduce the subsequent risk of fracture.

This was not the time, with so much at stake, for half measures. Merck planned and sponsored a massive two-pronged Fracture Intervention Trial involving 6500 women with 'low bone density' drawn from eleven clinical centres across the United States to determine alendronate's efficacy in both 'primary' and 'secondary' prevention. The first 'prong' of the trial, secondary prevention, compared the outcome in 2000 women who had already sustained a vertebral fracture characteristic of severe osteoporosis and who were allocated to receive either the drug or placebo. The outcome certainly appeared favourable, alendronate reducing the risk of both a further vertebral fracture and – more important still – a major fracture of the hip or wrist by almost half. With 300,000 people in the United States sustaining a hip fracture every year, this impressive result generated much publicity, the CBS reporter covering the press conference describing it as 'almost miraculous'. The reality – as shown in Table A1.1 – is rather more modest. Here we note that, overall, alendronate reduced the number and risk of fractures from 183 (18.2 per cent) to 139 (13.6 per cent). So it works. Focusing on the most serious fracture in clinical terms – that of the hip, with all its implications for the necessity to have a hip replacement operation – alendronate does indeed reduce the risk by half (2.2 per cent placebo, 1.1 per cent alendronate). But in absolute terms that equates to just 1.1 per cent fewer people sustaining a fracture (2.2 minus 1.1). Similar considerations apply to fractures of the wrist.

'There can be no denying the need to consider appropriate preventive measures,' noted public health doctor Adrian Phillips in a letter to the *Lancet* commenting on the results – but that minuscule 1.1 per cent absolute reduction in the risk of sustaining a hip fracture 'means that 300 people need to take

Table A1.1 The results of the Fracture Intervention Trial, 'secondary' prevention (for those who have already had a fracture)

	Women with at least one previous fracture			
Type of fracture	Placebo	Rate %	Alendronate	Rate %
Any clinical fracture	183	18.2	139	13.6
Hip	22	2.2	11	1.1
Wrist	41	4.1	22	2.2

medication for a year to prevent just one hip fracture'. He then calculated that, given the cost of alendronate, this worked out at £100,000 per fracture avoided – thirty times more than the cost of a hip replacement.

Dr Phillips's reservations about alendronate's true worth apply in even greater measure to 'primary' prevention, as revealed by the outcome – published two years later – of the second prong of the Fracture Intervention Trial, involving 4500 women with a low T-score but without a previous history of fracture. Here too, in relative terms, alendronate appeared to perform very well, reducing the overall risk of fracture by an impressive 12 per cent and hip fracture by 18 per cent. But, as shown in Table A1.2, that translates into an absolute benefit for hip fractures of just 0.2 per cent, while perplexingly those taking alendronate had a higher rate of fractures of the wrist. These results could always be finessed, but it began to look as if, for all Merck's therapeutic originality and prodigious experience in developing and marketing new drugs, alendronate would prove to be a damp squib. In the aftermath of its launch in 1996 (with the proprietary name Fosamax) it struggled to generate an annual revenue of £200 million.

Table A1.2 The results of the Fracture Intervention Trial, 'primary' prevention (for those who have not had a fracture)

Type of fracture	Placebo No. (%)	Alendronate No. (%)	Relative risk reduction	Absolute risk reduction
Any clinical fracture	312 (14.1)	272 (12.3)	−12%	−1.8%
Hip	24 (1.1)	19 (0.9)	−18%	−0.2%
Wrist	70 (3.2)	83 (3.7)	+15%	+0.5%

There might be little difficulty in encouraging doctors to prescribe alendronate for 'secondary' prevention in those who had already sustained a vertebral fracture, and who thus would be presumed to have osteoporosis of sufficient severity to warrant a 'bone-strengthening' drug. The potentially vastly larger market for 'primary' prevention in the legions of the fit and healthy was a different matter. Hormone replacement therapy seemed to be the much better (and more 'natural') option, not only protecting against fractures but with all those additional advantages of minimising the distressing subjective symptoms associated with the menopause. There was certainly little incentive for the millions already taking HRT to bother with the rigmarole of having a Dexa-scan to establish their T-score, so the potential market for 'primary' prevention was limited to those women who were reluctant to take HRT indefinitely – and men, for whom there was no alternative.

Here Merck confronted another obstacle – the considerable scepticism of several influential commentators as to whether those 'minus' T-scores could reliably predict the subsequent risk of fracture. 'It is probably not the case,' observed Professor

Terence Wilkin, in an article in the *British Medical Journal*, that (as claimed by the advocates of the WHO's 'somewhat arbitrary' definition) 'it is now possible to accurately determine with Dexa-scanning an individual's risk of fracture.' On the contrary, the main determinant by far was not bone density but age – with an incremental 44-fold increase in fracture rate between the ages of fifty-five and eighty to which, as shown in Figure A1.1, bone density makes only a trivial contribution. This, he notes, is an 'important observation' because it suggests that 'something very important in the ageing process influences fracture risk *independent* of bone density'. And thus independent too of the potential benefits of bone-strengthening drugs. Those 'very important' factors include, as already alluded to, all the features of ageing – frailty, poor eyesight, impaired balance – that predispose to a fall.

Merck made heroic efforts to escape this triple bind of competition from HRT, the disappointing results of the

Figure A1.1 The relative contribution of bone mineral density (below the dotted line) and age to the probability of hip fracture

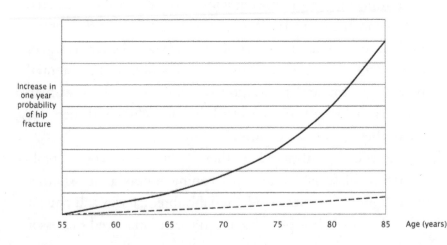

Increase in one year probability of hip fracture

55   60   65   70   75   80   85   Age (years)

primary prevention trials and the doubts as to whether bone density, as measured by the T-score, was a reliable guide to the subsequent risk of fractures, especially in oldies. Come 2002, prescriptions for Fosamax were only marginally higher than they had been six years earlier. But then came, as already described, the 'bombshell' – the publication of the Women's Health Initiative with its finding of the increased risk of breast cancer and the verdict that HRT probably 'did more harm than good'. HRT's fall from grace left the market wide open and Fosamax prescriptions took off like a rocket. In Britain over the next decade they would increase a staggering 45-fold, while worldwide sales by 2015 were generating, together with the several other bisphosphonates developed by Merck's competitors, £10 billion a year in revenue for their manufacturers. How did that happen, given the well-rehearsed arguments outlined above as to why the evidence for their efficacy seemed so underwhelming?

Doctors, no less than anyone else, are reluctant to acknowledge that they might have been wrong. They had, in good faith, extolled the virtues of HRT to their patients, not least in preventing fractures in later life, but now found themselves in the invidious situation of confronting the fact that on balance it might not be quite as terrific as they had portrayed. It was certainly a tricky situation, and the simplest way of resolving the dilemma was to propose some different bone-strengthening remedy, the singular virtue of Fosamax being precisely that it is 'a non-hormonal' drug and thus unencumbered by the adverse consequences associated with HRT.

Still, the switch from HRT to Fosamax could scarcely account for the continuous remorseless upward trend in prescriptions. Rather, doctors were encouraged to treat ever more patients by utilising a seductively simple, statistically based method for diagnosing osteoporosis known as the Fracture Risk Assessment Tool (FRAX), devised by none other than the chairman of the WHO committee, Professor John Kanis. This entails the family doctor typing in the relevant details of the patient's age, sex, and risk factors predisposing to bone fragility – smoking, alcohol consumption, family history of fractures, etc. Then up pops a coloured diagram in red and green illustrating the 'ten-year possibility of a major osteoporotic fracture'. Those whose score falls in the red area of the diagram warrant treatment with a bisphosphonate drug such as Fosamax. It could scarcely be simpler and does not even require the bother of having a Dexa-scan, though if the T-score is known this can be incorporated into the 'tool'.

FRAX is a big deal routinely used by doctors in forty countries, generating a million hits a day, many prescriptions for bisphosphonates and a considerable income for its copyright holder. It is thus of considerable interest to know how it was devised, and indeed how well it predicts those fractures that may (or may not) be prevented with medication. This, however, is not possible as the details have never been released. Numerous requests for clarification from research scientists and academics have drawn a blank. Dr Gary Collins of the University of Oxford comments:

'FRAX may have great potential, but it's debatable whether the scientific community has been provided with sufficient evidence to support its widespread use. This is compounded by the problem that FRAX is largely a *black box*, as the underlying equations behind them have never been placed in the public domain and it seems unlikely they will be published in the near future. It is unclear whether commercial and licensing issues are behind this but such secrecy makes it impossible for independent investigators to appropriately value and critique the model.'

Despite this aura of secrecy, FRAX has been incorporated into official 'guidelines'. For example, the *Clinician's Guide* published in the US by the National Osteoporosis Foundation in 2008 advised that anyone with a 3 per cent or greater ten-year possibility of sustaining a fractured hip warranted treatment. This almost doubled (from 6.4 to 10.8 million) those previously deemed eligible as determined solely by the T-score – to include 72 per cent of all women over the age of sixty-five. In Britain, the guidelines are slightly less ambitious, but the numbers in whom bisphosphonates are considered appropriate are substantial enough, ranging from 20 per cent of those aged fifty to 40 per cent of those aged eighty or older. Thus, one way or another the official endorsement of the FRAX 'diagnostic tool' accounts well enough for that exponential 45-fold increase in prescriptions.

And so to the flip side. While the vast majority of those taking bisphosphonates gain no advantage from doing so, all are vulnerable to the adverse effects they might cause. As journalist Cherrill Hicks wrote, describing her once-weekly ritual of taking Fosamax, 'I have come to dread the early morning ritual.' The requirement, after swallowing the tablet, to stay fully upright and neither eat or drink for thirty minutes is a necessary precaution against its tendency to cause inflammation of the lining of the oesophagus. Fosamax is not a pleasant drug to take, though the frequency of the more commonly cited side effects of nausea, dyspepsia and heartburn, as reported in the Fracture

Intervention Trial, was apparently 'not significantly higher than in those taking a placebo'. That claim would seem very unlikely.

Then, it subsequently emerged, the bisphosphonates possess the unusual property for a drug of causing precisely the problem – fractures – they are intended to prevent. In 2004, almost a decade after the launch of Fosamax, Dr Clarita Odvina of the University of Texas reported on nine patients, all taking bisphosphonates, who had sustained spontaneous fractures while 'performing normal daily activities such as walking or turning around'. Initially, if understandably, the connection had not been made, but when the fractures failed to heal in the normal manner, they all underwent a bone biopsy. This revealed 'markedly suppressed bone formation with minimal or no identification of osteoblasts'. The suggested explanation for this observation is as follows. The mechanism, as noted above, of the subtle relationship between the armies of bone-crunching osteoclasts and bone-forming osteoblasts in coordinating the cycles of remodelling remains unknown. Thus, it is possible that in some patients the inhibition, with bisphosphonates, of the osteoclasts might also suppress the osteoblasts (hence their apparent absence in the nine individuals tested). They are thus 'not available' to repair the microcracks that occur in bone due to the kind of stresses encountered in everyday life – resulting in those spontaneous stress fractures.

Several hundred further cases have been reported, accounting – according to a study conducted by orthopaedic surgeons in an Australian hospital – for around 5 per cent of the patients treated in the fracture clinic over a ten-year period. This might be classified as a 'rare' side effect. Rarer still is osteonecrosis of the jaw, where following dental extraction there is widespread destruction of bone, resulting in pain, swelling and recurrent infection that requires major reconstructive surgery. It is as grisly as it sounds. Merck initially denied liability, but in 2013 they paid $27 million in compensation to hundreds of those affected.

Fosamax undoubtedly works, increasing the bone density in those with osteoporosis and thus modestly reducing the subsequent risk of fracture. But, as with HRT, the question remains: on balance does it do more harm than good? The current situation would seem to be, if predictably, that bisphosphonates are of no value for 'primary' prevention; that is, for those who have not previously sustained a fracture or whose bone density scans are not seriously abnormal. 'They confer no proven clinically meaningful benefits in [reducing] hip or wrist fractures, most frequently associated with a diagnosis of osteoporosis.' As for 'secondary' prevention, for those who have previously had a fracture or a Dexa-scan with a T-score considerably less than –2.5, they will prevent a hip fracture in 1 per cent of those taking them and a vertebral fracture in one in twenty. There is, however, it now appears, little to be gained for this latter group in continuing treatment beyond five years.

'The current approach to preventing hip fractures with bisphosphonates is neither viable as a public health strategy nor cost-effective,' observed Professor Teppo Jarvinen of Helsinki University in the *British Medical Journal* in 2015. His analysis of twenty-three trials over the preceding years investigating the effectiveness of the drugs in preventing either primary or secondary hip fractures revealed that the vast edifice of Dexa-scanning, FRAX-determined diagnoses and mass prescribing was sustained by a difference of just thirty-five fewer hip fractures – the difference between the 254 out of 17,000 patients on treatment compared to 289 out of 14,000 'controls'. By his calculation, 175 people must take Fosamax, or its equivalent, for three years to prevent just one of them sustaining a hip fracture. This is, of course, desirable if you are that one lucky individual (though there is no way of determining if you might be) – but of no consolation to the remaining 174.

The crux of the matter, Professor Jarvinen maintains, is that fewer than one in three fractures can be reliably attributed to osteoporosis. Three-quarters of hip fractures occur in those aged seventy-five or over, for whom bone fragility may be a contributory factor but is vastly eclipsed by the increased risk of a fall. There is apparently no evidence from clinical trials that bisphosphonates specifically reduce the incidence of a fracture in this age group.

'This focus on drug treatment means that widely feasible non-pharmacological interventions are overlooked,' he argues – regular exercise, continuous monitoring of the effects of blood pressure-lowering drugs and sedatives that predispose to falls, and correcting 'hazards in the home' (such as poorly fitting carpets). To be sure, there remain some for whom bisphosphonates are certainly indicated, particularly those requiring long-term treatment with steroids or anti-cancer drugs that accelerate osteoporosis – but for most, 'They achieve at best a marginal benefit at the cost of unnecessary psychological harms, severe adverse events and forgotten opportunities to have a greater impact on the health of older people.' As such, their profligate prescription is 'an intellectual fallacy we will live to regret'.

This verdict elicited a sharp retort from the President of the International Osteoporosis Foundation (here encountered for the third time) Professor John Kanis. 'Professor Jarvinen's views are at odds with the overwhelming majority of his peers,' he wrote, and are 'inaccurate and misleading on a number of levels'.

Such as? 'There is strong evidence to demonstrate that drug treatment reduces fracture risk by 30–50%,' he added, though without clarifying what this means for the individual in absolute terms. Increasingly, however, it seems that doctors are coming to a rather different conclusion, signalled by a significant decline in bisphosphonate prescribing over the past few years.

Appendix 2

The (Toxic) Cardiac Cocktail

'Two years ago, I had a stent inserted following a heart attack. Prior to this I had been fully active in my retirement, visiting sites and fighting decisions on planning appeals. But since then I have been completely unable to work, spending much time resting and unable to concentrate on writing for more than half an hour. I suspect this disappointing outcome is attributable to one or more of the seven drugs I take. My consultants have made various amendments to my prescription, but with no success. If I were taking just one or two drugs, there would clearly be no difficulty in testing for damaging side effects. But identifying any harmful drugs in a group of seven or so is a problem. Has anyone developed a practical method of doing this?'

Mr D. H., building surveyor

The prospect for those admitted to hospital with a heart attack could scarcely be improved upon – tellingly illustrated by an incident when watching with a group of friends a performance of *King Lear* at the Old Vic with the legendary Glenda Jackson in the title role. Just twenty minutes in, one of the party started to feel very uncomfortable, sweating and shifting around in his seat – followed soon after by his having to leave. *King Lear*, at three and a half hours, is Shakespeare's longest play; still, it was astonishing to learn that by the time Glenda Jackson had taken her curtain call, my acquaintance having been admitted to nearby St Thomas' Hospital had already had a stent inserted to restore the blood flow to his blocked coronary artery.

Back in the 1950s, those admitted to St Thomas' with a heart attack would have been confined to bed for up to six weeks to allow the damaged muscle to heal – a major contributory factor (as will be seen) to the high mortality rate in those days where one-third of those who made it to hospital did not survive. For my acquaintance, back home within a couple of days, the probability of that terminal misfortune had fallen to just 2.5 per cent. That almost fifteen-fold improvement in the prospects of survival ranks among the great achievements of modern medicine. But, perversely one might think, for a substantial proportion of the 20,000 beneficiaries every year of percutaneous coronary intervention (PCI), as it is known, and the further 20,000 who require coronary bypass surgery, the quality of their lives is seriously compromised by the requirement to take a cocktail of drugs whose enervating adverse effects, as for the building surveyor cited at the opening of this chapter, had left him 'completely unable to work'.

There is, of course, a rationale for each of the five drugs that make up the standard cocktail – aspirin and an antiplatelet drug to thin the blood, a cholesterol-lowering statin (of course), a beta blocker and an ACE inhibitor to which may be added variously a diuretic, an acid suppressant and an antiarrhythmic drug. It would be a miracle if those on the cocktail did not experience one or more of its many potential adverse effects. One evening, when convalescing from a 'rather spectacular heart attack', Derrick Baxby, a former senior lecturer in microbiology at Liverpool University, took the opportunity to read the patient information leaflets on his battery of pills and totted them up. 'My seven tablets offered a choice of at least 130 side-effects', he observed in an article in the *British Medical Journal*. They fell, he noted, into three distinct categories. 'The first are relatively easy to recognise: impaired taste, hair loss, sexual dysfunction and sensitivity to sunlight.' It was more difficult to identify the culprit in the second group: 'Diarrhoea or constipation, runny or stuffy nose – all offered by carvedilol (beta blocker) and ramipril (ACE inhibitor) – and the former by frusemide, pravastatin and warfarin.' The third group were those side effects 'which can mimic or might be related to the underlying cardiac condition: slowed heartbeat (carvedilol and amiodarone), dizziness or low blood pressure (carvedilol, frusemide, ramipril), palpitations or chest pains (amiodarone, carvedilol, ramipril).' 'But how do I know which drugs are causing which side-effects,' he asks, 'as obviously there is considerable overlap. All may cause nausea and vomiting; five, rash or itching; five, diarrhoea or constipation; four, headache; four, chest pains or palpitations; and three, dizziness and low blood pressure. I will pass over the possibility that most may also cause kidney or liver problems – or both.'

The cocktail's considerable potential for causing iatrogenic illness must be offset, one would assume, by each drug's contribution to that fifteen-fold improvement in outcome following a heart attack. Thus, say drugs x, y and z each boosted the chances of survival by 20 per cent, then collectively that would add up to 60 per cent, which would be very worthwhile. This, however, is not necessarily the case. The studies needed to demonstrate that their individual contributions to improving survival are indeed 'additive' would require comparing the outcome with a similar group of patients taking a similar cocktail of placebo pills. This has never been attempted – nor will it be. Then again, it is highly probable that the wonders of PCI in promptly restoring blood flow to the heart muscle may well have trumped those additive benefits of taking drugs x, y and z – thus negating the need to take them. But, again, this has never been formally investigated.

Thus, those like my acquaintance find themselves in a most invidious situation. They are as grateful as anyone can be for their cardiologist's skilful and expeditious restoration of the blood flow to their heart muscle and, being naturally anxious to avoid a further episode, are readily persuaded to take the cocktail. But as time passes, the burden of taking so many pills becomes ever more onerous. For many, no doubt, they are a constant reminder of their mortality, compounded by fatigue or inertia or any of those other 130 side effects identified by Derrick Baxby – which, as he points out, can mimic precisely the cardiac symptoms (dizziness, palpitations, chest pains) they are intended to prevent.

Their cardiologists might be sympathetic to their plight but are, in general, persuaded by the merits of the cocktail, which have over time acquired the status of holy writ – endorsed by numerous national professional organisations and incorporated into their official guidelines. Thus, the standard response to those who might query, for any number of reasons, whether it is strictly necessary to 'keep on taking their pills' is that, on balance, they should do so. And there has, till recently, been no one to argue otherwise, until Professor Desmond Julian, Foundational Professor of Cardiology at Newcastle University – prompted by his own harrowing experiences – forcefully and authoritatively expressed a dissenting view.

Professor Julian is a luminary in the cardiac world, having instigated back in the 1960s a substantial improvement in survival by insisting that patients be admitted to a specialist coronary care unit to ensure that any potentially life-threatening disturbances of heart rhythm be properly diagnosed and treated. So, when he himself had the misfortune to have a heart attack, he had no hesitation about taking the standard cocktail of (as they are known) cardio-protective drugs. All went well for several years until he experienced three major side effects, starting with severe bleeding from the gut (aspirin), then a chronic intractable cough (the ACE inhibitor) and two near-death experiences, a precipitous fall in his blood pressure following exertion and collapse due to the slowing of his heart rate – both 'almost certainly' attributable to his beta blocker – that would have been fatal 'if immediate medical help had not been available'. Such potentially fatal episodes, he speculated, might well be 'not uncommon', prompting in turn his re-examination of the scientific evidence for the routine prescribing of the cardiac cocktail. From this he concluded that despite being prescribed to millions, its 'efficacy and safety are quite unknown' in the long term.

He suggests three main reasons as to how this situation has come about. The first is inappropriate (or false) extrapolation – where it is simply presumed that the evidence of the efficacy of, for example, beta blockers, based on clinical trials that run for just eighteen months, can be extrapolated to justify their 'open-ended administration over many years'. This is not at all certain. The risk of potentially fatal disturbances of heart rhythm, which those beta blockers are intended to protect against, is highest immediately following a heart attack, when the injured and inflamed heart muscle is most 'excitable', becoming progressively less so as it heals. Thus their efficacy will similarly diminish over time.

Next, the provenance of that 'evidence'. The findings from drug company-sponsored clinical trials employed to evaluate their merits is (for obvious reasons) not necessarily reliable, while at the same time militating against a proper evaluation of the several components of the cocktail. Put simply, the manufacturer of, for example, an ACE inhibitor need only demonstrate its efficacy in prolonging survival following a heart attack when compared to a placebo. Their ACE inhibitor can then be added to the 'cocktail', but the crucial question of its merits within the wider context of other cardio-protective drugs is not addressed. Thus, 'Newly licensed drugs are continually being introduced, whereas older drugs are not commonly reassessed – and therefore stay in use.'

Then there is the problem which almost did for Professor Julian himself. As time passes the body ages and its ability to handle drugs diminishes. They may cause no problems for a decade or more but then begin to do so, either on their own account or by interacting with the other components of the cocktail. Thus, ACE inhibitors may indeed have a modest beneficial effect, but they also increase the risk of sudden death by, for example, increasing the levels of potassium in the blood. Hence the paradox where drugs intended to prolong survival may shorten it – and no one would know. Had Professor Julian's potentially lethal beta blocker-induced near-death experiences occurred when alone, or in bed at night, his passing would have been attributed to anno domini. It was only because 'immediate help was available' that the true – iatrogenic – cause could be ascertained.

It is, of course, impossible to know how frequently this may occur. But Professor Julian's supposition that 'it is not uncommon' is no mere conjecture, informed as it is by historical precedent. Twice in his professional career, similarly widely endorsed treatments for heart disease, intended like the cardiac cocktail to prolong life, have had precisely the reverse effect. For several decades doctors insisted on a rigidly imposed regime of compulsory bed rest for up to three months following a heart attack, on the grounds that by protecting against the hazard of over-exertion, this would allow the heart muscle to heal. Just to read about it now is to be baffled that they could have been so blind to its devastating physical and mental consequences, aghast at the misery and suffering it must have caused. As the relevant passage in the 1950 edition of Frederick Price's influential *Textbook of the Practice of Medicine* reads:

'At least three months complete bed rest is indicated. After the patient has been confined to bed for two months, an extra pillow may be allowed, a week or so later the back of the bed may be gradually more raised, and during the last two weeks passive graduated exercises of the body and limbs, light massage and breathing exercises may be employed. After the period in bed, the patient should be moved to a couch to which he should be confined for at least two weeks. Then slight walking exercises may gradually be attempted. If, during any of these later stages, exertion be accompanied or followed by any abnormal symptoms, the amount of exertion has been too much and should be proportionately reduced.'

It is scarcely necessary to itemise the consequences, so obvious in retrospect, of this 'enforced recumbency' – pulmonary embolism, deep vein thrombosis, wasting of the leg muscles, loss of calcium from the bone, constipation, pneumonia, chronic invalidism and untimely death. 'Look at the patient lying long in bed, what a pathetic picture he makes!' wrote physician Richard Asher, a stern critic of this regime. 'The blood clotting in his veins, the lime draining from his bones, the faeces stacking up in his colon, the flesh rotting from his buttocks, the urine leaking from his distended bladder and the spirit evaporating from his soul.' The regime, it is subsequently estimated, would have been responsible for tens of thousands of 'unnecessary' deaths till its belated replacement in the 1960s by one of early mobilisation.

The second iatrogenic misfortune came twenty years later with the over-zealous promotion of drugs to suppress 'ventricular ectopic beats' – the intermittent perturbation of the pulse experienced as 'missed' beats – in the absence of any certain evidence of their efficacy.

These 'missed beats' are very common and harmless in themselves but following a heart attack might predispose, it was suggested, to life-threatening disturbances of heart rhythm. The introduction in the mid-1980s of two related drugs, flecainide and encainide, which successfully abolished these 'ventricular ectopics' led to the untested assumption that their routine use would reduce the risk of sudden unexpected death. But the trial (the Cardiac Arrhythmia Suppression Trial) intended to confirm this revealed the contrary, as within eighteen months there were almost three times more fatalities (sixty-three versus twenty-six) in those taking the drugs. Prescriptions plummeted, but their prior prescription, it would subsequently be alleged, may already have cost the lives of several thousand patients.

The relevance of these historical precedents of iatrogenic harm might seem at best tangential to current concerns, but parallels there certainly are. Cardiologists nowadays are no more likely to question the necessity of prescribing the cardiac cocktail following a heart attack or bypass surgery – sanctioned by many years of professional consensus – than their predecessors were to doubt the merits of prolonged bed rest sixty years ago. And this despite those serious 'gaps in knowledge' as to their efficacy to which Professor Julian draws attention, and of which indeed they might be unaware. And for the millions on the receiving end of the cocktail, the most significant 'gap' of all, the absence of any systematic investigation of the incidence, prevalence and severity of the side effects they might cause.

What then is to be done? Or, specifically, how can the building surveyor cited at the opening of this chapter extricate himself from the invidious situation – like those cardiac patients of sixty years ago – of 'having to spend much time resting and being quite unable to work'? Professor Julian proposes a series of measures: 'More rigorous monitoring of long-term drug use', 'Regular reviews to consider whether drugs might be discontinued', 'Better awareness of the need to avoid the trap of routine prescribing and the potential for side effects especially in the context of polypharmacy' – and so on. It is, however, one thing to identify the need for such measures; quite another for them to happen. This would seem unlikely, at least in the foreseeable future.

Thus, for those whose quality of life is seriously compromised there is really no other alternative than to take the initiative themselves and, by becoming acquainted with the merits and drawbacks of the main categories of cardio-protective drugs, create the opportunity to discuss with their doctor whether they wish to continue taking them indefinitely. This may not be popular, as querying medical advice is likely to elicit the brush-off, 'I would not be prescribing them if I did not think they were necessary.' So it is important to appreciate that doctors, especially general practitioners, are not conversant with the main points at issue as set out by Professor Julian and might welcome the opportunity for an informed discussion. In what follows I will consider in turn each of the main groups of drugs – the beta blockers, ACE inhibitors and statins – in relation to the specific questions that he raises: the nature of the evidence concerning their long-term use following a heart attack and their continuing relevance since the advent of PCI. This also provides the opportunity to consider the same questions as they apply to patients following bypass surgery.

Beta blockers

First introduced back in 1964, beta blockers retain their preeminent role fifty years later among the most widely prescribed class of drugs because of their manifold benefits, not just for those with one or other of the three main cardiac conditions – angina, hypertension and disturbances of heart rhythm – but, as will be seen, many others as well. The origins of this 'wonder drug' go back to the late 1940s, when American physiologist Raymond Ahlquist sought to resolve the fundamental problem of why the ubiquitous 'fight or flight' hormone, adrenalin, should have so many seemingly contradictory effects – both narrowing and dilating the blood vessels, constricting and widening the airways, stimulating and relaxing the muscles of the gut, bladder and uterus and increasing the rate and contractility of the heart muscle. These contradictory properties, he proposed, could best be accounted for if adrenalin's action were mediated by two different types of receptor (excitatory and inhibitory) that he labelled 'alpha and beta'. Thus, when one runs for a bus, for example, adrenalin's stimulatory action on the beta receptors causes the heart rate to increase, pumping more blood out into the circulation and down into the limbs. That rise in pulse rate also increases the heart's own need for oxygenated blood, which for those with the narrowed arteries of coronary heart disease cannot be fulfilled – a phenomenon experienced as the characteristic chest pain of angina. 'Blocking' the action of adrenalin on the beta receptors will prevent the pulse rate from rising, thus allowing those with heart disease to do more before the onset of their angina. And so, it turned out, very usefully and convincingly demonstrated in the study of the effects of the first beta blocker, propranolol, in just fourteen patients incapacitated by angina, reducing the frequency of their episodes of chest pain by more than two-thirds. Nor was that all: beta blockers also (quite unexpectedly) lowered the patients' blood pressure, leading to their use as a highly effective treatment for hypertension.

The 1960s was certainly a very fertile period of therapeutic innovation, but for a single drug to revolutionise the management of two such common and previously difficult-to-treat conditions was unprecedented – an achievement appropriately acknowledged by the award to their discoverer, Sir James Black, of the Nobel prize for medicine.

And as time passed, the therapeutic scope of the wonder drug expanded still further, being found to reduce the frequency and severity of migraine attacks, control the symptoms of an overactive thyroid (thyrotoxicosis), reduce the risk of blindness by lowering the pressure within the eyeball in patients with glaucoma and, very importantly, to provide an alternative to tranquillisers in suppressing the distressing palpitations and tremor associated with anxiety, panic attacks and stage fright. 'Beta blockers eliminate the physical impediment of musical performance caused by stage fright,' noted one report, 'significantly improving its quality as judged by music critics.'

By the late 1970s beta blockers were the most widely prescribed of any class of drug. And they would, their manufacturers hoped, become yet more profitable in their role as the first of the cardio-protective drugs prescribed to all following a heart attack in anticipation of prolonging survival. There were sound reasons for supposing they would do so. There are few more stressful situations than the crushing pain and doom-laden fear of a heart attack: the adrenalin levels soar, boosting the heart rate and thus the heart muscle's need for oxygenated blood, a need which – as the blood flow to the coronary arteries is obstructed – cannot be met. This in turn increases the scale of muscle damage, potentially precipitating the lethal disturbance of heart rhythm, ventricular fibrillation. The value of beta blockers administered during the first few hours in countering the harmful consequences of this adrenalin surge are self-evident. So, might their longer-term prescription be similarly beneficial?

The question has been investigated in no less than thirty-one clinical trials – an enormous multiplication of energy and expense brought about by each drug company's need to test its own brand of beta blocker for this indication. The findings are, however, remarkably consistent, as exemplified by the 1982 Betablocker Heart Attack Trial (BHAT) involving almost four thousand patients and lasting three years, at the end of which there were 27 per cent fewer deaths in those taking propranolol compared to placebo. Taken together with the (very similar) results of the thirty other trials, the verdict that 'Betablockers are effective in long-term prevention' provides the basis for the current recommendation that they be prescribed indefinitely. The legitimacy of this extrapolation must, however, be qualified by two familiar considerations. First, as always, the 'absolute' benefit for the individual is much more modest than the 27 per cent reduction in mortality would suggest. As shown in Table A2.1, the difference between the 9.8 per cent of those dying in the placebo group and the 7.2 per cent in those taking propranolol is just 2.6 per cent. Put another way, taking a beta blocker increases the chances of your being alive eighteen months later from 90.2 per cent to 92.8 per cent. This scarcely justifies, as Professor Julian observed, its long-term blanket prescribing to all.

Table A2.1 The results of treatment with beta blockers following a heart attack

Propranolol n = 1910		Placebo n = 1921	
No. of deaths	Rate %	No. of deaths	Rate %
138	7.2	188	9.8

And next, while the likelihood of any individual benefiting from taking beta blockers for this indication is modest, all are exposed to the risk of adverse effects from the undesirable consequences of blocking the excitatory action of adrenalin on those beta receptors. While the action of beta blockers in slowing the heart rate reduces the heart muscle's need for oxygen and thus the severity of anginal attacks, it inevitably compromises its pump-like action so that less blood is propelled into the circulation. This is experienced by some of those taking beta blockers as 'a loss of pep'; for others a state of chronic fatigue:

'I required a coronary angioplasty some years ago with the insertion of four stents since when I have been taking 5mg bisoprolol, amongst other medications. Since then I have suffered tiredness, fainting on aeroplanes and "not feeling very lively". Recently a locum GP sent me to see a kidney specialist because I was suffering from "extreme tiredness syndrome". She turned out to be a real star and took a holistic view recommending I purchase a blood pressure monitor and record the results for a few weeks before going to see my own GP about possibly revising my medication. I duly did this and found that sometimes my blood pressure was as low as 100 and my heart rate in the 50s. My GP agreed to reduce the bisoprolol to 2.5mg. After a few days, I started to feel much better and now feel significantly more "lively" (at least for a 71-year-old). I feel that for all these years my heart has been over controlled by the beta blocker and I have a much better balance between my quality of life and "protection".'

Furthermore, blocking the beta receptors elsewhere in the body results, variously, in cold extremities (by reducing the blood flow to the limbs), wheezing and shortness of breath (from narrowing the airways), a less fulfilling sex life for men (for obvious reasons) and, through their effect on the brain, nightmares, insomnia and low mood.

And then there is the possibility, illustrated by Professor Julian's near-death experiences, that beta blockers previously tolerated can become with time dramatically less so, producing a potentially fatal slowing of the heart rate and a precipitous fall in blood pressure on exertion.

ACE inhibitors

The concept of blocking adrenalin's excitatory effects on the beta receptors in the heart is relatively easy to grasp, and is certainly useful in understanding both how they might be 'cardio-protective' and how they might cause certain side effects. The same, regrettably, cannot be said for ACE inhibitors. Few know they even have an Angiotensin Converting Enzyme, let alone what it might do or why it might need 'inhibiting'.

The gist is as follows. The hormone angiotensin, secreted by the liver, fine-tunes the blood pressure in two distinctive ways, adjusting both the calibre of the blood vessels and the amount of salt and water passing through the kidneys. Thus, if the blood pressure falls for any reason, angiotensin counters this by constricting the blood vessels (as squeezing the end of a hosepipe increases the water pressure), and expanding the volume of fluid in the circulation by reducing the amount of salt and water excreted in the urine.

The role of the angiotensin-converting enzyme, as its name suggests, is that it converts the precursor of the hormone known as angiotensin I into its active form, angiotensin II. Thus, a drug that 'inhibits' this has the opposite effect to that just described, lowering the blood pressure in those with hypertension by dilating the blood vessels and increasing the volume of urine excreted. This latter 'diuretic effect' has the further benefit of relieving the breathlessness of patients with heart failure by shifting the 'fluid in the lungs'.

We are indebted for this most useful class of drug to the Brazilian pit viper *Bothrops jararaca*, 3ft (0.9m) long with striking zigzag markings and an aggressively protruding tongue. Endemic in the south-west of the country, it poses a particular hazard to workers on banana plantations who, when bitten, collapse from a drastic drop in their blood pressure. In the mid-1960s, a Brazilian research student arrived in London with a vial of the viper's venom in his back pocket that Sir John Vane, 'one of the greatest pharmacologists of the twentieth century', found contained a novel chemical responsible for that precipitous drop in blood pressure by inhibiting the action of the angiotensin-converting enzyme.

It was not immediately obvious that this fortuitous discovery from such an unlikely source could be turned to therapeutic advantage as a treatment for raised blood pressure, but the drug company E. R. Squibb persevered and in 1975 launched captopril – the first of many ACE inhibitors that proved to be not only very effective in lowering the blood pressure but remarkably well tolerated. Sir John Vane himself, when diagnosed with hypertension, naturally opted to be treated with a drug to whose development he had made such a significant contribution. He would be among the first to experience its commonest side effect, a chronic intractable cough.

The drug companies, seeking to 'grow the market' for their ACE inhibitors beyond treating hypertension and heart failure, hoped that, like propranolol, it would prove to be 'cardioprotective' for patients following a heart attack. Clinical trials investigating this possibility would be organised in three phases, starting with those with severe heart failure (and thus most likely to benefit from its 'diuretic' effect), then those with impaired functioning of the heart muscle, and finally those with 'stable' heart disease. In each category ACE inhibitors reduced the risk of dying (as with propranolol) by an impressive 25 per cent, relatively speaking, but in absolute terms this falls from a very useful 6.3 per cent in those with severe heart failure to just 1 per cent in those with stable heart disease.

There were sound commercial reasons for the drug manufacturers to organise the trials in this manner because with each phase the numbers involved rise exponentially. Those with heart failure (and thus most likely to benefit) are few, those with stable heart disease (and least likely to do so) are many. The constancy of that 'relative' figure of improving survival by around a quarter allowed the drug companies to promote their ACE inhibitors on the grounds that they are uniformly effective, thus legitimising their routine prescription. But for most, those with stable heart disease and least likely to benefit, the advantage is very small indeed.

The corollary that all are nonetheless exposed to the hazards of adverse effects matters less than with the beta blockers as ACE inhibitors are in general well tolerated. Around one in ten, like Sir John Vane, would develop a chronic cough, but this is a conspicuous and readily recognisable side effect correctable by discontinuing the drug. The more sinister side to the ACE inhibitors is that with time their diuretic properties, so useful in lowering the blood pressure and eliminating 'fluid on the lungs', disturbs the fluid and electrolyte balance in the body, causing the levels of potassium to rise and increasing the risk of acute kidney failure.

Around one in ten of those on ACE inhibitors have a raised level of potassium in the blood, which increases the excitability of the heart muscle predisposing to potentially serious disturbances of heart rhythm. Still, this is a routine finding and no cause for alarm. But other commonly prescribed drugs, such as the antibiotic cotrimoxazole and anti-inflammatory drugs, can also raise the potassium level and, in combination, their synergistic effect can be dangerous.

ACE inhibitors, too, are almost a masterclass in the dangers of polypharmacy in the older age group, many of whom will be taking non-steroidal anti-inflammatory drugs (NSAIDs) for their age-related aches and pains, as well as 'water pills'. The three taken together account for half of patients admitted to hospital with drug-induced kidney failure.

Statins

The chequered history behind the third ingredient of the cardiac cocktail, the cholesterol-lowering statins, is prescribed in Chapter 4. Their role in primary prevention when prescribed to the otherwise fit and healthy may be vigorously disputed, but there can be no doubting their value as cardio-protective drugs prolonging survival in those known to have heart disease. This is epitomised by the striking outcome of the 4S Trial that launched the statin project, with its 41 per cent (relative) and 3.6 per cent (absolute) reduction in cardiac mortality. Their beneficial effect may well be offset for those in whom they cause variously muscular aches and pains, low mood, loss of memory and general decrepitude – but this, too, has already been considered in some detail.

The statins are, however, unique in being the only one of the trio of cardio-protective drugs for which there is any evidence favouring their long-term prescription. Six years on, those taking pravastatin have clearly done better (see Table A2.2) – though not as significantly as in the 4S Trial – with 24 per cent (relative) and 1.9 per cent (absolute) fewer deaths from heart disease.

* * *

This epic journey through the gradual evolution of the cardiac cocktail from the BHAT Trial onwards has been a bit of a slog,

Table A2.2 The results of long-term treatment (seven years) with pravastatin following a heart attack

	Placebo (n=4502)		Pravastatin (n=4512)		Relative risk reduction	Absolute risk reduction
	No.	Rate %	No.	Rate %		
Cardiac death	373	(8.3)	281	(6.4)	−24%	−1.9%

but not without interest, while drawing attention to those 'gaps in knowledge' of the current practice of indefinite prescribing highlighted by Professor Julian. Each ingredient of the cocktail acts in a different way, so it would be reasonable to assume their combined effectiveness would be additive. That would mean, taken together, that in 'relative' terms they might prolong survival by a most impressive 76 per cent – beta blocker (27 per cent) plus ACE inhibitor (25 per cent) plus statin (24 per cent). Little wonder perhaps that patients can be so readily persuaded that the merits of these drugs outweigh their hazards. The 'absolute' benefit when combined ranges from 6 per cent in those with 'stable' heart disease to 12 per cent in those with complications such as heart failure – a lot more modest, certainly, than suggested by those relative figures, but many might still consider it worthwhile.

But then we confront the most significant 'gap in knowledge' of all, where that evidence of benefit is in a sense 'ancient history', trumped as it were by the dizzying technical achievement of PCI in promptly restoring blood flow to the injured heart muscle. Reperfusion has proved to be one of the most

Figure A2.1 The prompt restoration of blood flow with thrombolytic drugs or PCI has dramatically reduced the risk of dying following a heart attack

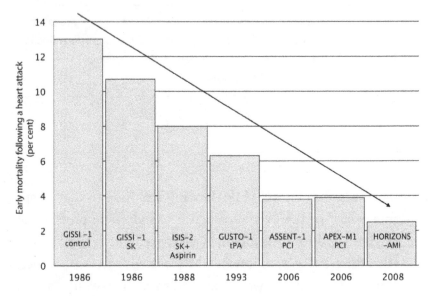

dramatically successful treatments of modern times, as vividly portrayed in Figure A2.1, which traces the downward trend in 'early mortality' following a heart attack over the past twenty years.

We start in 1986 with GISSI, an Italian trial involving 11,000 patients with a mortality rate of 13 per cent in the control group, falling to 10.7 per cent in those receiving the blood-thinning drug streptokinase (SK). Add in aspirin (the Isis Trial) and that figure falls to 8 per cent, while a more effective type of blood-thinning drug (the Gusto-1 Trial) reduces it again, to 6.3 per cent. Then with the advent of PCI (Assent), early mortality falls still further to 3.8 per cent, and finally in the Horizons Trial in 2008 to just 2.5 per cent.

Thus, the prompt restoration of blood flow, by limiting the

scale of injury to the heart muscle, makes a massive difference to the immediate outcome, and there is every reason to suppose that this should carry over favourably, influencing on a similar scale the long-term prognosis. And that would convincingly seem to be the case, for the outcome following PCI is now so good as to be little different from that of those without heart disease at all. Indeed, twelve years on, those who have undergone reperfusion are now more likely to succumb from non-cardiac causes (pneumonia, cancer, etc.) than heart disease. This almost unbelievably excellent long-term outcome leaves little scope for the cardiac cocktail to fulfil its 'protective' role. That would seem a common-sense inference but, regrettably, common sense counts for little in modern times where the only criteria of the truth are the hard data of clinical trials. The necessary clinical trial that would compare the cocktail with placebo will, however, never happen: hence the invidious situation of the building surveyor in the opening chapter, and so many like him:

'I had a heart attack last October and was treated at a London hospital and discharged on multiple dosages of several drugs. Since then I have noticed a persistent deterioration in my faculties – muscular aches, dizzy spells and the slowing down of both physical and mental abilities. The doctor insists I continue taking them – but I am very reluctant to do so.'

Now the way round this knowledge 'deficit' – in the absence of the relevant clinical trials – pioneered by Dr Sripal Bangalore of the New York University School of Medicine, would be to track the progress of large numbers (20,000 patients) and compare how well those taking beta blockers fared compared to those who did not. He subsequently carried out a similar exercise for ACE inhibitors and, as might be expected, for both it transpired that for those with stable heart disease it made no difference whether they were or were not taking either drug. By contrast, those on statins – as suggested by the pravastatin study mentioned above – do indeed modestly benefit from their protective effect over several years.

Professor Julian's concerns about the wisdom of indefinite prescribing do seem amply justified. The benefits of the cocktail, modest in the pre-perfusion era, are now much more modest still. There is every reason for those debilitated by the 'hangover' of its adverse effects to discuss with their doctors whether they would be better off by discontinuing some or all of the drugs – not least because of the chances, sooner or later, of 'running into trouble'.

* * *

The same considerations apply to the tens of thousands for whom the cocktail is routinely prescribed following bypass surgery and non-acute, or primary, coronary angioplasty. Both procedures avoid the inevitable hazards associated with any emergency intervention and so are considerably safer than PCI following a heart attack. Their outcomes are likely to be better still and the benefits of the cocktail commensurately more marginal.

It is difficult to be sure by how much, for here the rationale of prescribing this trio of cardio-protective drugs is based for the most part on no more than extrapolation – namely that, as they appear to confer benefit following a heart attack, they should do for similar reasons following bypass surgery. The questionable logic of such extrapolation has rarely been challenged – to the detriment unfortunately of many, as I am painfully reminded by the ordeal of a close friend whose wife's original idea for his sixty-fifth birthday present was to pay for a comprehensive medical check-up. He felt well enough but his exercise electrocardiogram was a bit iffy, leading him to have a coronary angiogram that revealed narrowing of two of his coronary arteries. Following his bypass surgery, he became severely depressed, a not unusual – if unexplained – complication that usually improves within six months. He did not. He had, he told me, become 'a zombie', which he attributed to his brain interpreting the fact that during his operation his heart was stopped (to perform the procedure) as meaning he must have died. He had joined the ranks of the living dead. Fanciful, perhaps, but that is how it felt. His enthusiasm for drawing and illustration, by which he earned his living, evaporated; he became a recluse wracked by suicidal thoughts. And so it continued for several years, not helped by his reluctance to seek or certainly take psychiatric advice. I suggested the culprit might be the statin he was taking and advised he discontinue it. When this made no difference I urged him to ask his cardiologist whether he might lay off the other two components of his cocktail, the beta blocker bisoprolol and the ACE inhibitor ramipril. His specialist reluctantly agreed, starting with the bisoprolol. A fortnight later he was 'a new man'. 'It is as if I have lost five years of my life,' he told me.

Inspired by his miraculous recovery, I reviewed the relevant 'literature'. This is how it looks.

Beta blockers

These reduce the risk of developing atrial fibrillation in the immediate post-operative period following bypass surgery and, following angioplasty, for six months. As for the longer term, their value following cardiac surgery ranges from none to a small absolute benefit (1.6 per cent) at four years. They confer no benefit following coronary angioplasty at three years.

ACE inhibitors

There is now general agreement that ACE inhibitors 'confer no benefit'.

Statins

Here the two relevant studies show that, seven years after bypass surgery, those taking a 'high' compared to a 'moderate' dose of lovastatin had 2.5 per cent fewer fatal and non-fatal heart attacks. Following coronary angioplasty, those taking statins had 2.2 per cent fewer heart attacks and 0.5 per cent fewer deaths at three years.

Epilogue

Dear Dr James,

I can attest to the miserable and devastating effects of [the cardiac cocktail]. I had a heart attack in June 2016. Best of hospital care, heart very happy with the new stent, no pain. I had not taken any prescription medication of any kind before this event. My only health complaint: osteoarthritis (knees).

On leaving hospital I was 'issued' with atorvastatin, bisoprolol, ramipril, clopidogrel and aspirin. I became sleepless, giddy, sweating day and night, disoriented and lost weight (which I didn't need to do). I felt as if I were going mad. After a couple of weeks, I went to my GP who fortunately is a listener. He took me off the atorvastatin and clopidogrel, saying they were 'the usual culprits' for the side effects I had given him. I persevered with the others for another six weeks of misery, then saw him again to tell him I was taking myself off the drugs. He told me, 'I have no problem with that!' My heart was happy and comfortable with its new 'runway' [the PCI]. All the drugs did was interfere with my recovery. I have to say that, give or take a dodgy episode now and then, I am back to my usual self.

Acknowledgements

This book, if obviously, could never have been written if not for all who over the past ten years have written to tell so graphically and compellingly of their personal experiences of too much medicine. Beyond words, thank you. I am indebted too to friends and colleagues whose encouragement and insights have been more important than they can realize: Fiona Godlee, Iona Heath, Malcolm Kendrick, Jerome Burne, Paula Byrne, Michael Fitzpatrick, Mark Ashworth, Jasper Mordhorst, Jenny Law, Jane Logan, Ray Moynihan, Margaret McCartney, Des Spence, Dee Mangin, John Yudkin, Klim Mcpherson, Richard Lehman and Carl Heneghan.

My heartfelt gratitude, as ever, to my splendid agent Caroline Dawnay, my publisher Richard Beswick and editor Tamsyn Berryman, to Caroline Sherbrooke for her prodigious secretarial skills and literally invaluable support and, beyond measure, to my wife Juliet.

Sources

Introduction

1   **In just fifteen years the number of prescriptions** ... Martin Beckford, 'Amount of drugs prescribed by GPs triples over 15 years', *Daily Telegraph,* 1 April, 2011.

1   **The *British Medical Journal,* among others** ... Ray Moynihan, 'Winding back the harms of too much medicine', *British Medical Journal,* 2013, Vol. 346, f1271; Deborah Grady, 'Less is More', *Archives of Internal Medicine,* 2010, Vol. 170 (No. 9), pp. 749-50; Margaret McCartney, 'Overdiagnosis and Overtreatment', *British Journal of General Practice,* 2016, pp. 110-117.

2   **The adverse consequences of 'polypharmacy'** ... D. A. Gorard, 'Escalating Polypharmacy', *Quarterly Journal of Medicine,* 2006, Vol. 99, pp. 797–800.

2   **And polypharmacy can also be fatal** ... Nigel Hawkes, 'The curious case of 600 extra deaths a week', *British Medical Journal,* 2013, Vol. 347, p. 15014.

2   **More than forty years ago, Henry Gadsden** ... W. Robertson, *Fortune,* March 1976.

2   **Ten years later a prominent British epidemiologist** ... Geoffrey Rose, 'Sick Individuals and Sick Populations', *International Journal of Epidemiology,* 1985, Vol. 14, pp. 32–38.

3   **In 2004, the long-standing contractual arrangements** ... S. Gillam, A. Niroshan Siriwardena, *The Quality and Outcomes Framework,* Radcliffe Publishing, 2011.

4   **There is, however, an historical precedent** ... Maurice Pappworth, *Human Guinea Pigs,* Routledge and Kegan Paul, 1967.

Chapter 1

7 Over the past sixty years, medicine has metamorphosed ... James Le Fanu, *The Rise and Fall of Modern Medicine*, Abacus, 2011.

7 And yet the more powerful and prestigious ... Peter Conrad, 'The Shifting Engines of Medicalization', *Journal of Health and Social Behavior*, 2005, Vol. 46, pp. 3–14.

8 In the very recent past the number of prescriptions ... Martin Beckford, 'Amount of drugs prescribed by GPs triples over 15 years', *Daily Telegraph*, 2011. See also D. A. Gorard, 'Escalating polypharmacy', *Quarterly Journal of Medicine*, 2006, Vol. 99, pp. 797–800. See also Bruce Guthrie, 'The rising tide of polypharmacy and drug-drug interactions: population database and analysis 1995–2010', *BMC Medicine*, 2015, Vol. 13 p. 74.

9 This widening of the scope of those deemed eligible ... Office of Health Economics, 'Compendium of Health Statistics', 2009; Health & Social Care Information Centre, 'Prescriptions Dispensed in the Community England 2003–13', 2014.

12 Whenever visiting the surgery nowadays ... Malcolm Kendrick, *Doctoring Data*, Columbus Publishing, 2014.

12 The biggest change over the course of my career ... Margaret McCartney, *The Patient Paradox*, Pinter & Martin, 2012.

14 The number of patients seriously injured ... P. F. D'Arcy, *Iatrogenic Diseases*, Oxford University Press, 1986.

21 Back in 1979, almost forty years ago ... Cedrick R. Martys, 'Adverse reactions to drugs in general practice', *British Medical Journal*, 1979, Vol. 2, pp. 1194–1197.

22 And then the trend reversed ... Nigel Hawkes, 'The curious case of 600 extra deaths a week', *British Medical Journal*, 2013, Vol. 347, p. 15014.

22 Several commentators have attributed it to 'austerity' ... Rachel Loopstra et al., 'Austerity and old-age mortality in England: a longitudinal cross-local area analysis, 2007–2013', *Journal of the Royal Society of Medicine*, 2016, Vol. 109 (3), pp. 109–116.

22 They include a woman in her nineties ... Ian Scott, 'Preventing Overdiagnosis', *Conference Barcelona*, 2016.

24 The insight that more than anything ... Ray Moynihan, *Selling Sickness*, Nation Books, 2005.

24 And so it has come about, as Marcia Angell observes ... Marcia Angell, *The Truth About the Drug Companies*, Random House, 2004.

25 It is, however, of interest to note here ... Peter C. Gotzsche, *Deadly Medicines and Organised Crime*, Radcliffe Publishing, 2013.

28 The first is a striking graph of the rise and fall ... Reuel Stallones, 'The Rise and Fall of Ischaemic Heart Disease', *Scientific American*, 1980, Vol. 243, pp. 43–9.

30 Most would readily agree to take a drug ... LRC-CPPT, 'Reduction in Incidence of Coronary Heart Disease', *Journal of the American Medical Association*, 1984, Vol. 251, pp. 351–73.

Chapter 2

34 On 12 April 1945 Roosevelt died ... Franz Messerli, 'This Day Fifty Years ago', *New England Journal of Medicine*, 1995, Vol. 332, pp. 1038–9.

36 In 1944 a German-born physician at Duke University ... Walter Kempner, 'Treatment of Hypertensive Vascular Disease with Rice Diet', *American Journal of Medicine*, 1948, Vol. 4, pp. 545–77.

37 The almost unbelievable benefit they confer ... Veterans' Administration Co-operative Study Group, 'Effects of Treatment on Morbidity in Hypertension', *Journal of the American Medical Association*, 1967, Vol. 202, pp. 1028–33.

39 Now, predictably the risk of stroke ... Prospective Studies Collaboration, 'Cholesterol, diastolic blood pressure, and stroke: 13,000 strokes in 450,000 in 45 prospective cohorts', *The Lancet*, 1995, Vol. 346, pp. 1647–53.

40 Come the end of the study ... Medical Research Council, 'MRC Trial of Mild Hypertension: Principal Results', *British Medical Journal*, 1985, Vol. 291, pp. 97–103.

42 Those adverse effects, sufficiently serious ... Medical Research Council, 'Adverse Reactions to Bendrofluazide and Propranolol for the Treatment of Mild Hypertension', *The Lancet*, 1981, Vol. 2, pp. 539–43.

42 This theory, first proposed by prominent epidemiologist ... Geoffrey Rose, 'Sick Individuals and Sick Populations', *International Journal of Epidemiology*, 1986, Vol. 14, pp. 32–8. See also Geoffrey Rose, 'The Population Mean Predicts the Number of Deviant Individuals', *British Medical Journal*, 1990, Vol. 301, pp. 1031–5; Geoffrey Rose, *The Strategy of Preventive Medicine*, Oxford: Oxford University Press, 1992.

46 But it is scarcely necessary to point out ... Bruce G. Charlton, 'A critique of Geoffrey Rose's "population strategy" for preventive medicine', *Journal of the Royal Society of Medicine*, 1995, Vol. 88, pp. 607–610.

46 The supposition that the 'average' blood pressure ... Peter Skrabenek, 'The mean predicts the number of deviants', *British Medical Journal*, 1990, Vol. 301, p. 1394.

47   Twenty years later another prominent epidemiologist ... Michael
      Marmot, *Rose's Strategy of Preventive Medicine*, Oxford University Press,
      2008.

48   **My blood pressure was recorded as 154/78 ...** Oscar M. Jolobe, 'Mild
      hypertension in people at low risk', *British Medical Journal*, 2014, Vol.
      349, f5432.

48   **We have two options in dealing with the massive number of patients ...**
      Edmund A. Willis, 'NHS health checks and QOF increase overtreat-
      ment', *British Medical Journal*, 2012, Vol. 345, e6172.

49   **It is all too often that a hospital doctor sees patients ...** Jecko Thachil,
      'Can I stop my blood pressure tablets?', *British Medical Journal*, 2010,
      Vol. 341, c4102.

50   **Indeed, when informed consent is sought ...** David Misselbrook,
      'Patients' responses to risk information about the benefits of treating
      hypertension', *British Journal of General Practice*, 2001, Vol. 51, pp.
      276–279.

50   **The further reason it is necessary for doctors to seek ...** S. J. Jachuck
      et al., 'The effect of hypotensive drugs on the quality of life', *Journal of
      the Royal College of General Practitioners*, 1982, Vol. 32, pp. 103–105.

50   **The side effects of the more commonly prescribed ...** Y. Trinder,
      'Common and less common adverse effects of antihypertensives', *South
      African Family Practice Journal*, 2012, Vol. 54 (2), (Suppl. 1), pp. S31–S32.

53   **To take just one example, from Canada ...** Brenda R. Hemmelgarn,
      'Trends in antihypertensive drug prescriptions and physician visits in
      Canada between 1996 and 2006', *Canadian Journal of Cardiology*, 2008,
      Vol. 24, pp. 507–512.

53   **The definitive verdict came in 2012 ...** Stephen A. Martin, 'Mild
      hypertension in people at low risk', *British Medical Journal*, 2014, Vol.
      349, g5432.

Chapter 3

58   **The novelty of this epidemic of coronary disease ...** Maurice Cassidy,
      'Coronary Disease: The Harveian Oration', *The Lancet*, 1946, Vol. 2, pp.
      587–90.

58   **On the contrary, the first description in Britain ...** J. W. McNee, 'The
      Clinical Syndrome of Thrombosis of the Coronary Arteries', *Quarterly
      Journal of Medicine*, 1925, pp. 44–51.

59   **First it was necessary to know more about the predisposing ...** Ancel
      Keys et al., 'Mortality and Coronary Heart Disease Among Men

Studied for Twenty-three Years', *Archives of Internal Medicine*, 1971, Vol. 128, pp. 201–14. See also Ancel Keys et al., 'The CVD Research Programme of the Laboratory of Physiological Hygiene: The Journal', *The Lancet*, 1961, pp. 291–5.

60   It remained a puzzle until ... Ancel Keys, 'From Naples to Seven Countries: A Sentimental Journey', *Progress in Biochemical Pharmacology*, 1983, Vol. 19, p. 130.

60   Over the next few years Keys travelled the world ... Ancel Keys et al., 'Lessons from Serum Cholesterol Studies in Japan, Hawaii and Los Angeles', *Annals of Internal Medicine*, 1958, pp. 83–93; Ancel Keys, 'Coronary Heart Disease in Seven Countries', *Circulation*, 1970, Vol. 41, Suppl. 1, pp. 1–211.

64   First, it failed to account for the very striking ... Reuel Stallones, 'The Rise and Fall of Ischaemic Heart Disease', *Scientific American*, 1980, Vol. 243, pp. 43–9.

64   Yet even though their dietary pattern remains ... J. Cornfield & S. Mitchell, 'Selected Risk Factors in Coronary Disease', *Archives of Environmental Health*, 1969, Vol. 19, pp. 382–94.

64   As one of his critics, Sir George Pickering ... George Pickering, 'Pathogenesis of Myocardial Infarction', *British Medical Journal*, 1964, pp. 517–29.

66   A subtle point, perhaps but sometimes subtlety ... Irvine H. Page et al., 'Atherosclerosis and the Fat Content of the Diet', *Circulation*, 1957, Vol. 16, pp. 163–78.

66   In 1957, at the time of the publication ... Jeremiah Stamler et al., 'Diet and Serum Lipids in Atherosclerotic Coronary Heart Disease', *Medical Clinics of North America*, 1963, Vol. 47, pp. 3–28.

67   Its next report, predictably, was very different ... 'Ad Hoc Committee on Dietary Fat and Atherosclerosis; Dietary Fat and its Relation to Heart Attack and Strokes', *Circulation*, 1961, Vol. 23, pp. 133–6.

69   They were then randomly allocated into either ... Mr Fit Research Group, 'Multiple-risk Factor Intervention Trial', *Journal of the American Medical Association*, 1982, Vol. 248, pp. 1465–77.

70   Hence the interest in the second of the two studies ... World Health Organisation European Collaborative Group, 'Multi-factorial Trial in Prevention of Heart Disease Incidence and Mortality Results', *European Heart Journal*, 1983, Vol. 4, pp. 141–7.

71   Clearly this was impossible ... James Le Fanu, *The Rise and Fall of Modern Medicine*, Abacus, 2011. See also *WHO Health Statistics Annual, 1952–84*, World Health Organisation, Geneva. See also *FAO Production*

Yearbook, 1982, Food and Agriculture Organisation, Rome.

74 **From 1982 to 1987 seven different reports** ... G. Cannon and C. Walker, *The Food Scandal,* Century, 1984.

74 **The omission from these reports of any explanation** ... J. R. A. Mitchell, 'What constitutes evidence in the dietary prevention of Coronary Heart Disease? Cosy beliefs or harsh facts?', *International Journal of Cardiology,* 1984, Vol. 4, p. 287.

76 **As for the second interested party** ... LRC-CPPT, 'Reduction in Incidence of Coronary Heart Disease', *Journal of the American Medical Association,* 1984, Vol. 251, pp. 351–73. See also Editorial, 'Is Reduction of Blood Cholesterol Effective?'.

80 **And sure enough, in December 1984** ... Consensus Conference, 'Lowering Blood Cholesterol to Prevent Heart Disease', *Journal of the American Medical Association,* 1985, Vol. 253, pp. 2080–7. See also 'Campaign Seeks to Increase US Cholesterol Consciousness', *Journal of the American Medical Association,* 1986, Vol. 255, pp. 1097–1102.

83 **In 1992, Dr Chochuo Kuo of the University of Washington** ... A. Shor et al., 'Detection of Chlamydia in Coronary Arterial Fatty Streaks and Atheromatous Plaques', *South African Medical Journal,* 1992, Vol. 82, pp. 158–61.

83 **Dr Stephen Epstein, also of the University of Washington** ... S. Epstein, 'The Multiple Mechanisms by which Infection May Contribute to Atherosclerosis Development and Course', *Circulation Research,* 2002, Vol. 90, pp. 2–4.

Chapter 4

85 **In 1976 Henry Gadsden** ... W. Robertson, *Fortune,* March 1976.

86 **Some idea of the extraordinary scale** ... James Le Fanu, *The Rise and Fall of Modern Medicine,* Abacus, 2011.

86 **There was 'A Dearth of New Drugs'** ... Editorial, 'A Dearth of New Drugs', *Nature,* 1980, Vol. 283, pp. 609. See also Fred Steward and George Wibberley, 'Drug Innovation: What's Slowing it Down? *Nature,* 1980, Vol. 284, pp. 118–20; Richard J. Wurtman and Robert L. Bettiker, 'The Slowing of Treatment Discovery, 1965–95', *Nature Medicine,* 1995, Vol. 1, pp. 1122–5.

87 **This sharp decline in the numbers of new drugs** ... A. Willman, 'Thalidomide and Foetal Abnormalities', *British Medical Journal,* 1962, p. 477. See also Editorial, 'Thalidomide's Long Shadow', *British Medical Journal,* 1976, pp. 1155–6.

87 **But the 'dearth of new drugs'** ... Jack W. Scannell, 'Diagnosing the decline in pharmaceutical R&D efficiency', *Nature Reviews Drug Discovery*, 2012, Vol. 11, pp. 191–200.

90 **If the industry was to have a viable future** ... Jeremy A. Greene, *Prescribing by Numbers: Drugs and the Definition of Disease*, The John Hopkins University Press, Baltimore, 2007.

91 **Akira Endo speculated that antibiotics** ... Thomas P. Stossel, 'The Discovery of Statins', *Cell*, 2008, Vol. 134, pp. 903–6.

93 **Our primary effort will be devoted to** ... 'Cholesterol Breakthrough: Mevacor Caps a Decades-Long Research Effort', *Merck World 8*, 1987, Vol. 5, pp. 4–13.

94 **'It used to be that the drug companies** ... Marcia Angell, *The Truth About the Drug Companies: How They Deceive Us and What to Do about It*, Random House, 2004.

95 **In his best-selling critique of the industry** ... Ben Goldacre, *Bad Pharma: How Drug Companies Mislead Doctors and Harm Patients*, Fourth Estate, London, 2012.

95 **The first is for 'primary prevention'** ... J. Shepherd et al., for the West of Scotland Coronary Prevention Study Group. 'Prevention of coronary heart disease in men with hypercholesterolemia', *New England Journal of Medicine*, 1996, Vol. 333, pp. 1301–1307.

96 **The next is 'secondary' prevention** ... J. Kjekshus, for the Scandinavian Simvastatin Survival Study Group. 'Reducing the risk of coronary events: evidence from the Scandinavian simvastatin survival study (4S)', *American Journal of Cardiology*, 1995, Vol. 76, pp. 64–80.

96 **Soon afterwards, the experts decreed** ... H. Gilbert Welch, Lisa M. Schwartz, Steven Woloshin, *Overdiagnosed: Making People Sick in the Pursuit of Health*, Beacon Press, Boston, 2011.

97 **'By the end of the 1990s** ... Jeremy A. Greene, *Prescribing by Numbers: Drugs and the Definition of Disease*, The John Hopkins University Press, Baltimore, 2007.

98 **But what does this actually mean** ... John-Arne Skolbekken, 'Communicating the risk reduction achieved by cholesterol reducing drugs', *British Medical Journal*, 1998, Vol. 316, pp. 1956–8. See also David M. Diamond and Uffe Ravnskov, *Expert Review of Clinical Pharmacology*, 2015, Vol. 8(2), pp. 201–210.

100 **Hence the catchily titled PROSPER trial** ... J. Shepherd et al., 'Pravastatin in elderly individuals at risk of vascular disease (PROSPER): a randomised controlled trial', *The Lancet*, 2002, Vol. 360, pp. 1623–30.

103 'As a rheumatologist, my job is to help people ... Andrew Bamji, 'Viewpoint: The hidden (and painful) cost of statins', *Daily Mail*, 27 January 2009. See also Andrew Bamji, 'Adverse effects of statins', *British Medical Journal*, 2014, Vol. 348, g3306.

107 Thus, a survey of almost 8000 French statin users ... E. Bruckert, G. Hayem, S. Dejager, C. Yau, B. Bégaud, 'Mild to moderate muscular symptoms with high-dosage statin therapy in hyperlipidemic patients – the PRIMO study', *Cardiovascular Drugs and Therapy*, 2005, Vol. 19 (6), pp. 403–14.

108 Researchers scrutinising the medical records ... D. Gaist, 'Statins and risk of polyneuropathy', *Neurology*, 2002, Vol. 58 no. 9, pp. 1333–1337.

108 A search of the US Food and Drug Administration's database ... Duane Graveline, *Lipitor: Thief of Memory*, Six Star Publishing, 2004. See also Duane Graveline, 'Adverse Effects of Statin Drugs: a Physician Patient's Perspective', *Journal of American Physicians and Surgeons*, 2015, Vol. 20, pp. 7–11.

108 This was more than mere 'association' ... Beatrice A. Golomb, 'Statin-Associated Adverse Cognitive Effects: Survey Results from 171 Patients', *Pharmacotherapy*, 2009, Vol. 29 (7), pp. 800–811.

109 In 2012 the most prominent advocate of all ... Jenny Hope, 'Give statins to all over-50s: Even the healthy should take heart drug, says British expert', *Daily Mail*, 28 August 2012.

109 Soon after the publication of that first trial ... 'CTT: Cholesterol Treatment Trialists' Collaboration', www.ctsu.ox.ac.uk/research.

110 How costly is not known ... Zoë Harcombe, '*The Lancet* Statin Study', www.zoeharcombe.com/2016/09/the-lancet-statin-study, 2016.

110 Statins, it transpired, in a review published in 2012 ... Cholesterol Treatment Trialists' (CTT) Collaborators, 'The effects of lowering LDL cholesterol with statin therapy in people at low risk of vascular disease: meta-analysis of individual data from 27 randomised trials', *The Lancet*, 2012, Vol. 380, pp. 581–90. See also Shah Ebrahim, 'Statins for all by the age of 50 years?', *The Lancet*, 2012, Vol. 380, pp. 545–547.

110 This verdict, noted one of Professor Collins's collaborators ... Jonathan Wood, 'Statins for the many?', www.ox.ac.uk/media/science_blog/120517.html, 2012. Retrieved 13/09/2012.

110 Soon after publication of these rather astonishing findings ... Margaret McCartney, 'Statins for all?', *British Medical Journal*, 2012, Vol. 345, e6044.

112 'The observed risk [of heart disease] at ten years ... Julia Hippisley-Cox et al., 'Predicting cardiovascular risk in England and Wales: prospective

derivation and validation of QRISK2', *British Medical Journal*, 2008, Vol. 336, a332.

114 **They are not what they are cracked up to be** ... John Abramson et al., 'Should people at low risk of cardiovascular disease take a statin?', *British Medical Journal*, 2013, Vol. 347, f6123. See also J. Abramson, J. M. Wright, 'Are lipid-lowering guidelines evidence-based?', *The Lancet*, 2007, Vol. 369, pp. 168–9.

115 **'Questions about statins continue to emerge** ... Fiona Godlee, 'Lessons from the controversy over statins', *The Lancet*, 2017, Vol. 389, pp. 1100–1.

115 **'Saturated fats are not associated with coronary heart disease** ... Russell J. de Souza et al., 'Intake of saturated and trans unsaturated fatty acids and risk of all cause mortality, cardiovascular disease, and type 2 diabetes: systematic review and meta-analysis of observational studies', *British Medical Journal*, 2015, Vol. 351, h3978.

115 **Next, it transpired that the 'coronary risk score'** ... S. Jamal, 'Accuracy of the Atherosclerotic Cardiovascular Risk Equation in a Large Contemporary, Multiethnic Population', *Journal of the American College of Cardiology*, 2016, DOI:10.1016/j.jacc.2016.02.055.

115 **Finally, the striking pattern of the 'rise and fall'** ... 'Deaths registered by cause, gender and age', *England and Wales, Office for National Statistics*, 2016 and 'Prescriptions Dispensed in the Community, England 2003–13, *Health & Social Care Information Centre*.

116 **We have here two pie charts** ... Michael Brooks, 'Cholesterol Wars', *New Scientist*, 2017, 11 March, pp. 29–33; David Newman, 'Statins Given for 5 Years for Heart Disease Prevention', *The NNT Group*, 2010–2018.

Chapter 5

123 **And very effective it is too** ... William Banting, *Letter on Corpulence*, 1864.

125 **The merit of the LCHF diet for those with Type 2 diabetes** ... D. R. Hadden et al., 'Maturity Onset Diabetes Mellitus: Response to Intensive Dietary Management', *British Medical Journal*, 1975, Vol. 3, pp. 276–278.

125 **This brings us to the conundrum posed** ... L. S. Geiss et al., 'Prevalence and incidence trends for diagnosed diabetes among adults aged 20 to 79 years, United States, 1980–2012', *Journal of the American Medical Association*, 2014, Vol. 312, pp. 1218–26. See also A. Hauber, 'The market in diabetes', *Diabetologia*, 2006, Vol. 49, pp. 247–252.

127   We start with the now familiar technique ... L. M. Schwartz and S. Woloshin, 'Changing Disease Definitions: Implications on Disease Prevalence', *Effective Clinical Practice*, 1999, Vol. 2, pp. 76–85.

127   In 2011 the diagnostic criterion was switched ... Nitin N. Gholap et al., 'Diagnosing type 2 diabetes and identifying high-risk individuals using the new glycated haemoglobin (HbA1c) criteria', *British Journal of General Practice*, February 2013, pp. 105–6.

127   Family doctors applying this new criterion ... Philip H. Evans, 'Diagnosing type 2 diabetes and identifying high-risk individuals using the new glycated haemoglobin (HbA1c) criteria', *British Journal of General Practice*, May 2013, pp. 235–6. See also Jonathan Sleath, 'In pursuit of normoglycaemia', *British Journal of General Practice*, July 2015, pp. 334–5.

127   Still, the almost quadrupling of the numbers diagnosed ... Dang M. Nguyen, 'The Epidemiology of Obesity', *Gastroenterology Clinics of North America*, March 2010, Vol. 39 (1), pp. 1–7.

128   In one of the most remarkable turnabouts in the history of medicine ... British Diabetic Association's Medical Advisory Committee Nutrition Sub-Committee. Dietary recommendations for the 1980s – A policy statement by the British Diabetic Association, *Human Nutrition, Applied Nutrition*, 1982, Vol. 36, pp. 378–86.

132   And the more drugs taken ... Dr. H. Gilbert Welch, Dr. Lisa M. Schwartz, Dr. Steven Woloshin, *Overdiagnosed*, Beacon Press, Boston, 2011.

133   The epidemiologists invoked the 'population approach' ... Simon Griffin et al., 'New QOF glycaemia targets are achievable and based on a balanced review of available evidence', *British Medical Journal*, 2009, Vol. 338, b800.

133   Meanwhile the pharmaceutical industry ... A. Hauber, 'The market in diabetes', *Diabetologia*, 2006, Vol. 49, pp. 247–252.

134   Theoretically it should ... Richard Lehman et al., 'Tight control of blood glucose in long standing type 2 diabetes', *British Medical Journal*, 2009, Vol. 338, b800. See also J. S. Yudkin et al., 'Intensified glucose lowering in type 2 diabetes: time for a reappraisal', *Diabetologia*, DOI:10.1007/s00125–010–1864–z; Bianca Hammingsen et al., 'Intensive glycaemic control for patients with type 2 diabetes: systematic review with meta-analysis and trial sequential analysis of randomised clinical trials', *British Medical Journal*, 2011, Vol. 343, d6898; Rozalina G. McCoy et al., 'Intensive Treatment and Severe Hypoglycemia Among Adults With Type 2 Diabetes', *Journal of the American Medical*

Association Internal Medicine, 2016, 176 (7), 969–978.

135 **The first, no more than a simpler version** ... Guenther Boden et al., 'Effect of a Low-Carbohydrate Diet on Appetite, Blood Glucose Levels, and Insulin Resistance in Obese Patients with Type 2 Diabetes', *Annals of Internal Medicine,* 2006, Vol. 142, pp. 403–411.

136 **Soon after, Dr Richard Feinman** ... Jeff S. Volek and Richard D. Feinman, 'Carbohydrate restriction improves the features of Metabolic Syndrome. Metabolic Syndrome may be defined by the response to carbohydrate restriction', *Nutrition & Metabolism,* 2005, Vol. 2, p. 31.

136 www.Diabetes.co.uk

136 **The majority feel the support they receive** ... Roberta Bernardi, *The Role of Online Health Communities in Patient Empowerment,* Royal Holloway University of London, September 2017.

137 **Eight months later they had lost on average a stone** ... Dr David Unwin, Dr Jen Unwin, 'Low carbohydrate diet to achieve weight loss and improve HbA1c in type 2 diabetes and pre-diabetes: experience from one general practice', *Practical Diabetes,* Vol. 31. No. 2.

138 **'Carbohydrate restriction is the first approach** ... Richard D. Feinman Ph.D., 'Dietary carbohydrate restriction as the first approach in diabetes management: Critical review and evidence base', *Nutrition,* 2015, Vol. 31, pp. 1–13.

139 **Epilogue: A master class in deprescribing** ... David Unwin, Simon Tobin, 'A patient request for some "deprescribing"', *British Medical Journal,* 2015, 351, h4023.

Chapter 6

144 **'That shared experience'** ... Iona Heath, *The Mystery of General Practice,* The Nuffield Provincial Hospitals Trust, 1995.

144 **That 'mutual bond of trust and respect'** ... Rachel Adam, '"Personal Care" and General Practice Medicine in the UK: A qualitative interview study with patients and General Practitioners', *Osteopathic Medicine and Primary Care,* 2007, Vol. 1, pp. 13. See also Carolyn Tarrant et al., 'Qualitative study of the meaning of personal care in general practice', *British Medical Journal,* 2003, 3:26: 1310–9.

146 **It all started, seemingly innocently enough** ... Martin Roland, 'Where did the Quality and Outcomes Framework come from?' in S. Gillam and A. Niroshan Siriwardena (Eds), *The Quality and Outcomes Framework,* Radcliffe Publishing, 2011. See also Nicholas Watt, 'Blair's £12bn pledge to NHS', *Guardian,* 17 January 2000.

147 'I entered General Practice in 1972 ... Dr Eric Rose, 'The True History of GP Out of Hours Services', https://abetternhs.net/2013/05/10/true-history.

151 This, 'the boldest proposal to improve ... Paul Shekelle, 'New contract for general practitioners', *British Medical Journal*, 2003, Vol. 326, pp. 457–8.

152 'The profession is being bribed ... Toby Lipman, 'Into the Sunlit Uplands?', *British Journal of General Practice*, May 2005, p. 396.

152 'I am increasingly dismayed ... Dougal J. Jeffries, 'A fresh new contract for general practitioners', *British Medical Journal*, 2002, 324: 1048.

153 A sensible decision as it turned out ... John Carvel, 'GP practices earning 58% more for 5% less work, audit office finds', *Guardian*, 28 February 2008.

153 The new contract, costed in anticipation ... National Audit Office, 'NHS Pay Modernisation: New Contracts for General Practice Services in England', The Stationary Office, London, 2008.

154 There was professional satisfaction ... Pooja Vaghela et al., 'Population Intermediate Outcomes of Diabetes Under Pay-for-Performance Incentives in England From 2004 to 2008', *Diabetes Care*, March 2009, Vol. 32, pp. 427–429. See also C. R. Simpson, 'Impact of the pay-for-performance contract and the management of hypertension in Scottish primary care', *British Journal of General Practice*, July 2011, e443.

154 Satisfaction too in their patients being so much better ... Ruth McDonald et al., 'Impact of financial incentives on clinical autonomy and internal motivation in primary care: ethnographic study', *British Medical Journal*, 2007, DOI:10.1136/bmj.39238.890810.BE.

155 Why was it, wondered Welsh GP ... Jonathan Richards, 'Is there an elephant in the room?', *British Journal of General Practice*, May 2009, pp. 376–7.

156 'We gain £1800 by omitting 110 poorly controlled patients ... Alistair Revolta, 'The New Contract: Quality, Money and Perverse Incentives', *British Medical Journal*, 2003, 326:457.

157 It is however much more sensible ... Edmund A. Willis, 'NHS health checks and QOF increase overtreatment', *British Medical Journal*, 2012, 345: e6172.

157 'The QOF is deeply corrosive ... Dee Mangin, 'The Quality and Outcomes Framework: what have you done to yourselves?', *British Journal of General Practice*, June 2007, pp. 435–7.

158 Two months later, a couple of epidemiologists ... Iona Heath, Julia Hippisley-Cox and Liam Smeeth, 'Measuring performance and

missing the point?', *British Medical Journal*, 2007, Vol. 335, pp. 1075–7.

158 **Hang on a minute** ... Martin Roland, 'The Quality and Outcomes Framework', *British Journal of General Practice*, July 2007, pp. 525–6.

159 **I have asked many people over the years** ... Charlotte Williamson, 'Secrecy and Coercion in the QOF: a scandal averted?', *British Journal of General Practice*, https://doi.org/10.3399/bjgp17X690977.

159 **None of those interviewed in a patient survey** ... Kerin L. Hannon et al., 'Patients' views of pay for performance in primary care: a qualitative study', *British Journal of General Practice*, 2012, 62 (598): e322–e328.

160 **Surely not – but tragically only too true** ... Armando H. Norman et al., 'The Quality and Outcomes Framework: Body commodification in UK general practice', *Social Science & Medicine*, 170 (2016) 77e86.

162 **In 2006 the government introduced** ... Naheed Mukadam et al., 'Diagnostic rates and treatment of dementia before and after launch of a national dementia policy: an observational study using English national databases', *British Medical Journal Open*, 2014, 4:e004119. DOI:10.1136/bmjopen–2013–004119.

165 **'They come to the surgery because they are feeling tired** ... Iain Crinson, 'How ready is general practice to improve quality in chronic kidney disease?', *British Journal of General Practice*, June 2010, pp. 401–5.

166 **'To be honest, it did scare me** ... Timothy Ellam, 'Chronic kidney disease in elderly people: disease or disease label?', *British Medical Journal*, 2015: 351: h6559.

167 **There was a quantum leap** ... Evangelos Kontopantelis et al., 'Recorded quality of primary care for patients with diabetes in England before and after the introduction of a financial incentive scheme: a longitudinal observational study', *British Medical Journal Quality and Safety*, 2013; 22:53–64.

168 **The pursuit of those QOF targets** ... N. Gallagher et al., 'Increase in the pharmacological management of Type 2 diabetes with pay-for-performance in primary care in the UK', *Diabetic Medicine*, DOI:10.1111/dme.12575.

170 **Meanwhile, as also described** ... Richard Lehman, 'Tight control of blood glucose in long standing type 2 diabetes', *British Medical Journal*, 2009; 338: b800.

170 **It was a similar story** ... Umme Alman et al., 'Statin induced diabetes and its clinical implications', *Journal of Pharmacology and Pharmacotherapeutics*, 2014 July–September; 5(3): 181–185. See also Yu-Hung Chang, Ming-Chia Hsieh, Cheng-Yuan Wang, Kun-Cheng Lin and Yau-Jiunn Lee, 'Reassessing the Benefits of Statins in the

Prevention of Cardiovascular Disease in Diabetic Patients – A Systematic Review and Meta-Analysis', *The Review of Diabetic Studies*, DOI:10.1900/RDS.2013.10.157.

171 **The number of referrals and admissions** ... Mark J. Harrison et al., 'Effect of a national primary care pay for performance scheme on emergency hospital admissions for ambulatory care sensitive conditions: controlled longitudinal study', *British Medical Journal*, 2014; 349: g6423.

171 **Next, the health gap between the social classes** ... Evangelos Kontopantelis et al., 'Investigating the relationship between quality of primary care and premature mortality in England: a spatial whole-population study', *British Medical Journal*, 2015; 350: h904.

171 **Finally, the prospect of saving** ... Andrew M. Ryan et al., 'Long-term evidence for the effect of pay-for-performance in primary care on mortality in the UK: a population study', *The Lancet*, 2016; 388: 268–74. See also Grant Russell, 'Does paying for performance in primary care save lives?', *British Medical Journal*, 2015; 350: h1051.

172 **To summarise, according to** ... Lindsay Forbes, 'Review of the Quality and Outcomes Framework in England', *Policy Research Unit in Commissioning and the Healthcare System*, December 2016.

172 **The QOF simply hasn't worked** ... Des Spence, 'Kill the QOF', *British Medical Journal*, 2013; 346: f1498.

173 **Epilogue: Ten commandments** ... Richard Lehman et al., 'Ten Commandments for patient-centred treatment', *British Journal of General Practice*, 2015; 65 (639): 532–533.

Chapter 7

176 **'Any drug that is worth using** ... R. Laurence, P. N. Bennett, *Clinical Pharmacology*, Churchill Livingstone, 1987.

176 **'Between 1995 and 2010** ... Bruce Guthrie et al., 'The rising tide of polypharmacy and drug-drug interactions: population database analysis 1995–2010', *BMC Medicine*, 2015, Vol. 13, pp. 74.

177 **'There were major increases in recorded prevalence** ... David Melzer et al., 'Much more medicine for the oldest old: trends in UK electronic clinical records', *Age and Ageing*, 2015, Vol. 44, pp. 46–53.

177 **'Between 1999 and 2008 the annual hospital admissions** ... Tai-Yin Wu et al., 'Ten-year trends in hospital admissions for adverse drug reactions in England 1999–2009', *Journal of the Royal Society of Medicine*, 2010, Vol. 103, pp. 239–250.

178 **'The figures are fairly sensational** ... Nigel Hawkes, 'The curious case

of 600 extra deaths a week', *British Medical Journal*, 2013; 347: f5014.

179 **A felicitous outcome indeed** ... Doron Garfinkel et al., 'The War against Polypharmacy: A New Cost-Effective Geriatric-Palliative Approach for Improving Drug Therapy in Disabled Elderly People', *Israel Medical Association Journal*, 2007; 9: 430–434.

179 **Three years later he repeated the exercise** ... Doron Garfinkel, MD; Derelie Mangin, 'Feasibility Study of a Systematic Approach for Discontinuation of Multiple Medications in Older Adults', *Archives of Internal Medicine*, October 11, 2010, Vol. 170 (No. 18), pp. 1648–54.

180 **It is not as if they fail to acknowledge** ... Alex Matthews-King, 'GPs are "overdiagnosing and overtreating older patients"', *Pulse* , 30 April 2014.

181 **Put simply, oldies are less equipped** ... P. A. Routledge et al., 'Adverse drug reactions in elderly patients', *British Journal of Clinical Pharmacology*, 2003, 57:1, 121–126. See also Lisa Nolan, 'Prescribing for the Elderly', *Journal of the American Geriatrics Society*, 1988, 36: 142–149. See also Umesh T. Kadam, 'Potential health impacts of multiple drug prescribing for older people', *British Journal of General Practice*, 2011; 61: 128–130.

181 **That apart, there is a long list** ... Denis O'Mahony, 'Inappropriate prescribing in the older population: need for new criteria', *Age and Ageing*, 2008, Vol. 37, pp. 138–141.

181 **Thus, an investigation of the factors** ... Marie-Laure Laroche et al., 'Is inappropriate medication use a major cause of adverse drug reactions in the elderly', *British Journal Clinical Pharmacology*, 2006, Vol. 63:1, pp. 177–186.

182 **How often does this happen?** ... Ingeborg K. Björkman, 'Drug-Drug Interactions in the Elderly', *The Annals of Pharmacotherapy*, 2002, Vol. 36, pp. 1675.

183 **Or, as professor of medicine Paula Rachon** ... Paula A. Rochon, Jerry H. Gurwitz, 'Optimising drug treatment for elderly people: the prescribing cascade', *British Medical Journal*, 1997, 315: 1096–9.

183 **But on top of this enhanced risk, crucially, the cumulative effects** ... Bhavik M. Shah, Emily R. Hajjar, 'Polypharmacy, Adverse Drug Reactions, and Geriatric Syndromes', *Clinics in Geriatric Medicine*, 2012, pp. 172–186. See also Oscar A. Cepeda and John E. Morley, 'Polypharmacy, is this Another Disease?', *Principles and Practice of Geriatric Medicine, 4th Edition*, 2006, John Wiley & Sons Ltd.

186 **Consider, for example, a woman** ... Cynthia M. Boyd et al., 'Clinical Practice Guidelines and Quality of Care for Older Patients

With Multiple Comorbid Diseases', *Journal of the American Medical Association*, August 10, 2005, Vol. 294, pp. 716–24.

188 **This brings us to the central unifying ...** H. Coulson, P. Prescott-Clarke, 'Health Survey for England 1994', HMSO 1996. See also Gitanjali M. Singh et al., 'The age associations of blood pressure, cholesterol and glucose: analysis of health examination surveys from international populations', *Circulation*, 2012 May 8; 125 (18): 2204–2211.

190 **He knows (or should know) ...** Richard A. Kronmal et al., 'Total Serum Cholesterol Levels and Mortality Risk as a Function of Age', *Archives of Internal Medicine*, 1993; 153: 1065–1073. See also Irwin J. Schatz, MD, 'Cholesterol and all-cause mortality in elderly Heart Program: a cohort study', *The Lancet*, 2001, Vol. 358, pp. 351–355.

191 **'Mr O, a bachelor farmer ...** George A. Sarosi, MD, 'The Tyranny of Guidelines', *Annals of Internal Medicine*, 2015, 163: 562–563.

195 **'Despite their wide-spread use ...** Michelle C. Odden et al., 'Cost-Effectiveness and Population Impact of Statins for Primary Prevention in Adults Aged 75 Years or Older in the United States', *American College of Physicians*, 2015, 162, pp. 533–41.

195 **Specifically, the merits of statins ...** J. Shepherd et al., 'Pravastatin in elderly individuals at risk of vascular disease (PROSPER): a randomised controlled trial', *The Lancet*, 2002; 360: 1623–30.

195 **As for diabetes, statins have ...** Jill P. Crandall et al., 'Statin use and risk of developing diabetes: results from the Diabetes Prevention Program', *British Medical Journal Open Diabetes Research and Care*, 2017; 5: e000438. See also Yu-Hung Chang, 'Reassessing the Benefits of Statins in the Prevention of Cardiovascular Disease in Diabetic Patients – A Systematic Review and Meta-Analysis', *The Review of Diabetic Studies*, DOI:10.1900/RDS.2013.10.157.

197 **The suspicion that those high systolic pressures ...** SHEP Cooperative Research Group, 'Prevention of stroke by anti-hypertensive drug treatment in older persons with isolated systolic hypertension: Final results of the Systolic Hypertension in the Elderly Program (SHEP)', *Journal of the American Medical Association*, 1991, 265: 3255–3264.

199 **Hence, as geriatrician Dr John Morley observes ...** John E. Morley, MB, BCh, 'Hypertension: Is It Overtreated in the Elderly?', *Journal of the American Medical Directors Association*, DOI:10.1016/j.jamda.2009.12.081.

199 **Falls, it is scarcely necessary to point out ...** Mary E. Tinetti et al., 'Antihypertensive Medications and Serious Fall Injuries in a Nationally Representative Sample of Older Adults', *Journal of the American Medical Association Internal Medicine*, 2014; 174(4): 588–595. See also Debra A.

Butt, 'The Risk of Hip Fracture After Initiating Antihypertensive Drugs in the Elderly', *Archives of Internal Medicine*, 2012; 172: 1739–1744.

201 **Regrettably these are not** ... J. S. Yudkin et al., 'Intensified glucose lowering in type 2 diabetes: time for a reappraisal', *Diabetologia*, 5 August 2010, DOI:10.1007/s00125–010–1864–z. See also Kasia J. Lipska, 'Potential Overtreatment of Diabetes Mellitus in Older Adults With Tight Glycemic Control', *Journal of the American Medical Association Internal Medicine*, 2015; 175(3): 356–362.

202 **So, from 2004 onwards** ... Francesco Zaccardi et al., 'Trends in hospital admissions for hypoglycaemia in England: a retrospective, observational study', *The Lancet Diabetes and Endocrinology*, August 2016, Vol. 4, No. 8, pp. 677–685.

202 **The low blood sugar or hypoglycaemia** ... J. E. Signorovitch et al., 'Hypoglycaemia and accident risk in people with type 2 diabetes mellitus treated with non-insulin antidiabetes drugs', *Diabetes, Obesity and Metabolism*, 2013, 15: 335–341. See also Philip E. Cryer, 'Severe Hypoglycemia Predicts Mortality in Diabetes', *Diabetes Care*, 2012, Vol. 35, pp. 1814–5.

202 **They would be avoided** ... Etie Moghissi, 'Management of Type 2 Diabetes Mellitus in Older Patients: Current and Emerging Treatment Options', *Diabetes Therapy*, 2013, 4: 239–256.

203 **Instead now the *lower* they are** ... Uffe Ravnskov, 'Lack of an association or an inverse association between low-density-lipoprotein cholesterol and mortality in the elderly: a systematic review', *British Medical Journal Open,* 2016; 6: e010401. See also Kari Mattila, MD, 'Blood pressure and five year survival in the very old', *British Medical Journal*, 26 March 1988, Vol. 296, pp. 887–890.

203 **Thus, logically, such prescriptions** ... Jean S. Kutner et al., 'Safety and Benefit of Discontinuing Statin Therapy in the Setting of Advanced, Life-Limiting Illness. A randomized Clinical Trial', *Journal of the American Medical Association Internal Medicine*, 2015; 175 (5): 691–700 ; Line Kirkeby Petersen et al., 'Lipid-lowering treatment to the end? A review of observational studies and RCTs on cholesterol and mortality in 80+-year olds', *Age and Ageing*, 2010, Vol. 39, pp. 674–680; Yvonne Morrissey et al., 'Older people remain on blood pressure agents despite being hypotensive resulting in increased mortality and hospital admission', *Age and Ageing*, 2016, Vol. 45, pp. 783–788; Wilbert S. Aronow, MD, 'Multiple Blood Pressure Medications and Mortality Among Elderly Individuals', *Journal of the American Medical Association Internal Medicine*, DOI:10.1001/jamainternmed.2014.8012.

Chapter 8

205 'There are many reasons why ... David P. Alldred, 'Deprescribing: a brave new word?', *International Journal of Pharmacy Practice*, 2014, Vol. 22, pp. 2–3.

206 The guiding principle for 'rolling back the harms' ... Richard Smith, 'Too much medicine? Almost certainly', *British Medical Journal*, Vol. 324, pp. 859–860.

206 Dr Ian Scott of the University of Queensland ... Ian Scott, 'Physicians need to take the lead in deprescribing', *Internal Medicine Journal*, 2015, Vol. 45, pp. 352–356. See also Nagham J. Ailabouni, 'Challenges and Enablers of Deprescribing: A General Practitioner Perspective', *PLOS ONE*, 2016, DOI:10.1371/journal.pone.0151066.

207 For all that, when 90 per cent of those ... Alex Matthews-King, 'GPs are "overdiagnosing and overtreating older patients"', *Pulse*, 30 April 2014.

209 The only other essential resource ... 'A practical guide to Stopping Medicines in Older People', *Best Practice Journal*, 2010, Issue 27, www.bpac.org.nz. See also Murthy Gokula et al., 'Tools to Reduce Polypharmacy', *Clinics in Geriatric Medicine*, 2012, 28, pp. 323–341; Jesse Jansen et al., 'Too much medicine in older people? Deprescribing through shared decision making', *British Medical Journal*, 2016, 353: i2893. See also Polly Duncan, 'Deprescribing: a primary care perspective', *European Journal of Hospital Pharmacy*, 2017, 24, pp. 37–42.

211 The scope for deprescribing ... Stephen A. Martin et al., 'Mild hypertension in people at low risk', *British Medical Journal*, 2014; 349: g5432. See also Jack Froom et al., 'Withdrawal of Antihypertensive Medications', *Journal of the American Board of Family Practice*, 1997, 10, 249–58.

211 For one in ten (or more) ... Malcolm Aylett et al., 'Stopping drug treatment of hypertension: experience in 18 British general practices', *British Journal of General Practice*, 1999, Vol. 49, pp. 977–980. See also T. Ekbom, 'A 5-year prospective, observational study of the withdrawal of antihypertensive treatment in elderly people', *Journal of Internal Medicine*, 1994: 235: 581–588.

212 Here the scope for deprescribing ... John D Abramson et al., 'Should people at low risk of cardiovascular disease take a statin?', *British Medical Journal*, 2013, 347: f6123. See also Timo E. Strandberg et al., 'Care of the Aging Patient: From Evidence to Action', *Journal of the American Medical Association*, 2014, 312, pp. 1136–1144; Jean S. Kutzner, 'Safety and Benefit of Discontinuing Statin Therapy in the Setting

of Advanced, Life-Limiting Illness. A Randomized Clinical Trial', *Journal of the American Medical Association Internal Medicine*, 2015, 175 (5), 691–700.

212 **The score, as recently noted** ... Jamal S. Rana, 'Accuracy of the Atherosclerotic Cardiovascular Risk Equation in a Large Contemporary, Multiethnic Population', *Journal of the American College of Cardiology*, 2016, 67, 2118.

212 **There is less scope for deprescribing** ... Dr David Unwin, 'Low carbohydrate diet to achieve weight loss and improve HbA1c in type 2 diabetes and pre-diabetes: experience from one general practice', *Practical Diabetes*, 2014, Vol. 31 (2): 1–4. See also D. R. Hadden, 'Maturity Onset Diabetes Mellitus: Response to Intensive Dietary Management', *British Medical Journal*, 1975, 3, 276–278.

213 *Polypharmacy is the disease* ... Doron Garfinkel, 'Routine deprescribing of chronic medications to combat polypharmacy', *Therapeutic Advances in Drug Safety*, 2015, Vol. 6, pp. 212–233.

213 **The options for deprescribing** ... Ian A. Scott, 'Reducing Inappropriate Polypharmacy. The Process of Deprescribing', *Journal of the American Medical Association Internal Medicine*, May 2015, Vol. 175 (5). See also Michael C. Woodward, 'Deprescribing: Achieving Better Health Outcomes for Older People Through Reducing Mediations', *Journal of Pharmacy Practice and Research*, 2003, 33, pp. 323–8.

213 **Here the practicalities are best illustrated** ... Cynthia M. Boyd et al., 'Clinical Practice Guidelines and Quality of Care for Older Patients With Multiple Comorbid Diseases', *Journal of the American Medical Association*, August 10, 2005, 294, pp. 716–724.

215 **When the previously mentioned Dr Ian Scott** ... Ian A. Scott, 'A medication review and deprescribing method for hospitalised older patients receiving multiple medications', *Internal Medicine Journal*, 2015, DOI:10.1111/imj.12906.

215 **The scope for improving** ... Doron Garfinkel, 'Feasibility Study of a systematic Approach for Discontinuation of Multiple Medications in Older Adults', *Archives of Internal Medicine*, 2010, 170 (18), pp. 1648–1654. See also Amy T. Page et al., 'The feasibility and effect of deprescribing in older adults on mortality and health: a systematic review and meta-analysis', *British Journal of Clinical Pharmacology*, 2016, 82, pp. 583–623.

216 **There is a memorable, if disturbing symmetry** ... Nigel Hawkes, 'The curious case of 600 extra deaths a week', *British Medical Journal*, 2013; 347: f5014.

Appendix 1

220 'She first notices weakness ... Gerald N. Grob, *Aging Bones: A short History of Osteoporosis*, Johns Hopkins University Press, Baltimore, 2014, p. 38.

221 And indeed it did ... Lila E. Nachtigall, 'Estrogen Replacement Therapy 1: A 10-Year Prospective Study in the Relationship to Osteoporosis', *Obstetrics and Gynecology*, 1979, Vol. 53, pp. 277–81.

222 That possibility of harm was ... Women's Health Initiative Investigators, 'Risks and Benefits of Estrogen Plus Progestin in Healthy Postmenopausal Women', *(Reprinted) Journal of the American Medical Association*, July 17, 2002, Vol. 288 (3), pp. 321–33.

223 'Ultimately it was just a matter of ... Alix Spiegal, 'How A Bone Disease Grew To Fit The Prescription', NPR.org, December 21, 2009.

223 The report of the meeting ... J.A. Kanis and the WHO Study Group, *Osteoporosis International*, 1994, Vol. 4, pp. 368–381. See also WHO Technical Report Series, 'Assessment of Fracture Risk and its Application to Screening for Postmenopausal Osteoporosis', *World Health Organization*, Geneva 1994.

225 The first 'prong' of the trial ... Dennis M. Black et al., 'Randomised trial of effect of alendronate on risk of fracture in women with existing vertebral fractures', *The Lancet*, 1996, Vol. 348, pp. 1535–41.

225 'There can be no denying ... Adrian Phillips, 'The Fracture Intervention Trial', *The Lancet*, 1997, Vol. 349.

226 Dr Phillips's reservations ... Steven R. Cummings et al., 'Effect of Alendronate on Risk of Fracture in Women With Low Bone Density but Without Vertebral Fractures', *Journal of the American Medical Association*, 1998; 280: 2077–2082.

227 'It is probably not the case ... Terence J. Wilkin, 'Changing perceptions in osteoporosis', *British Medical Journal*, 1999; 318: 862–5.

228 On the contrary, the main determinant ... Teppo L. N. Järvinen et al., 'Overdiagnosis of bone fragility in the quest to prevent hip fracture', *British Medical Journal*, 2015; 350: h2088.

229 In Britain over the next decade ... Tai-Yin Wu et al., 'Bisphosphonates prescription in England: 1996–2008', *British Medical Journal*, 2010; 341: c4444.

229 Rather, doctors were encouraged ... J.A. Kanis et al., 'Interpretation and use of FRAX in clinical practice', *Osteoporos International*, 2011, 22: 2395–2411.

230 'FRAX may have great potential ... Gary S. Collins, 'Fracture Risk Assessment: State of the Art, Methodologically Unsound, or Poorly

Reported?', *Current Osteoporosis Reports*, 2012, 10: 199–207. See also Teppo L. N. Järvinen MD PhD, 'Conflicts at the heart of the FRAX tool', *Canadian Medical Association Journal*, 2014, 186, p. 165.

231 **For example, the *Clinician's Guide* ...** Teppo L. N. Järvinen et al., 'Overdiagnosis of bone fragility in the quest to prevent hip fracture', *British Medical Journal*, 2015; 350: h2088.

232 **In 2004, almost a decade ...** Clarita V. Odvina et al., 'Severely Suppressed Bone Turnover: A Potential Complication of Alendronate Therapy', *The Journal of Clinical Endocrinology and Metabolism*, 2005, 90 (3), pp. 1294–1301.

233 **It is as grisly as it sounds ...** Nate Raymond, 'Merck agrees to proposed $27.7 million settlement over Fosamax lawsuits', *Reuters*, December 9, 2013.

233 **The current situation would seem to be ...** David Newman, 'Bisphosphonates for Fracture Prevention in Post-Menopausal Women Without Prior Fractures', *The NNT Group*, 2010–18.

233 **There is, however, it now appears ...** Dennis M. Black, Ph.D, 'Continuing Bisphosphonate Treatment for Osteoporosis – For Whom and for How Long?', *New England Journal of Medicine*, 2012, 366; 22: 2051.

233 **'The current approach to preventing ...** Teppo L. N. Järvinen et al., 'Overdiagnosis of bone fragility in the quest to prevent hip fracture', *British Medical Journal*, 2015; 350: h2088.

234 **This verdict elicited a sharp retort ...** Professor John A. Kanis, 'Overdiagnosis of bone fragility in the quest to prevent hip fracture', *British Medical Journal*, 2015; 350: h2088.

Appendix 2

239 **One evening, when convalescing ...** Derek Baxby, 'Is ignorance bliss?', *British Medical Journal*, 2001; 322: 872.

241 **All went well for several years ...** Xavier Rossello, Desmond Julian, 'Long-Term Use of Cardiovascular Drugs', *Journal of the American College of Cardiology*, 2015; 66: 1273–85. See also Desmond G. Julian, 'Effects of long-term use of cardiovascular drugs', *The Lancet*, 2015, Vol. 385, p. 325.

243 **As the relevant passage in the 1950 edition ...** Frederick Price (Ed.), *A Textbook of the Practice of Medicine*, Oxford University Press, 1950.

244 **'Look at the patient lying long ...** 'Richard Asher Talking Sense', *Pitman Medical*, 1979.

244 **But the trial** … Debra S. Echt et al., 'Mortality and Morbidity in Patients Receiving Encainide, Flecainide, or Placebo', *New England Journal of Medicine*, 1991; 324: 781–8.

244 **Prescriptions plummeted** … Thomas J. Moore, *Deadly Medicine: Why Tens of Thousands of Heart Patients Died in America's Worst Drug Disaster*, New York, Simon and Schuster, 1995.

247 **And so, it turned out** … P.M.S. Gillam, 'Use of Propranolol in Angina Pectoris', *British Medical Journal*, August 1965, 2, 337–8.

248 **The findings are, however** … BHAT Research Group, 'A Randomized Trial of Propranolol in Patients With Acute Myocardial Infarction', *Journal of the American Medical Association*, March 26, 1982, Vol. 247 (12), pp. 1707–14. See also Nick Freemantle, 'Beta Blockade after myocardial infarction: systematic review and meta regression analysis', *British Medical Journal*, 26 June 1999, Vol. 318, pp. 1730–7.

249 **While the action of beta blockers in slowing the heart rate** … William H. Frishman, 'β-Adrenergic Receptor Blockers: Adverse Effects and Drug Interactions', *Hypertension II (Suppl. II):II–21–II–29*, 1988. See also Mark H. Pollack et al., 'Propranolol and Depression Revisited', *The Journal of Nervous and Mental Disease*, Vol. 173, pp. 118.

252 **It was not immediately obvious** … David W. Cushman and Miguel A. Ondetti, 'History of the Design of Captopril and Related Inhibitors of Angiotensin Converting Enzyme', *Hypertension*, 1991, Vol. 17, pp. 589–593.

252 **Clinical trials investigating** … The Consensus Trial Study Group, 'Effects of Enalapril on Mortality in Severe Congestive Heart Failure', *New England Journal of Medicine*, 1987; 316: 1429–35; Marc A. Pfeffer et al., 'Effect of Captopril on Mortality and Morbidity in Patients with Left Ventricular Dysfunction after Myocardial Infarction', *New England Journal of Medicine*, 1992; 327: 669–77; Salim Yusuf et al., 'Effects of an Angiotensin-Converting-Enzyme Inhibitor, Ramipril, on Cardiovascular Events in High-Risk Patients', *New England Journal of Medicine*, 2000; 342: 145–53; Roberto Latini et al., 'ACE Inhibitor Use in Patients With Myocardial Infarction: Summary of Evidence From Clinical Trials', *Circulation*, 15 November 1995, Vol. 92 (10), pp. 3132–3137.

253 **But other commonly prescribed drugs** … Michael Fralick et al., 'Co-trimoxazole and sudden death in patients receiving inhibitors of renin-angiotensin system: population based study', *British Medical Journal*, 2014; 349: g6196. See also Merlin C. Thomas, 'Diuretics, ACE inhibitors and NSAIDs – the triple whammy', *Medical Journal of Australia*, 2000; 172:

184–5; Laurie A. Tomlinson, 'ACE Inhibitor and Angiotensin Receptor-II Antagonist Prescribing and Hospital Admissions with Acute Kidney Injury: A Longitudinal Ecological Study', *PLOS ONE*, 8(11): e78465.

254 **This is epitomised by ...** Terje Pedersen et al., 'Randomised trial of cholesterol lowering in 4444 patients with coronary heart disease: the Scandinavian Survival Study (4S)', *The Lancet*, 1994; 344: 1383–9.

254 **Six years on ...** LIPID Study Group, 'Prevention of Cardiovascular Events and Death with Pravastatin in Patients with Coronary Heart Disease and a Broad Range of Initial Cholesterol Levels', *New England Journal of Medicine*, 1998; 339: 1349–57.

255 **Reperfusion has proved to be ...** Frans Van de Werf, 'The history of coronary reperfusion', *European Heart Journal*, 2014, 35.2510–2515.

257 **And that would convincingly seem ...** Frants Pedersen et al., 'Short- and Long-Term Cause of Death in Patients Treated With Primary PCI for STEMI', *Journal of the American College of Cardiology*, 2014, Vol. 64: 2101–8.

257 **Now the way round this knowledge 'deficit' ...** Sripal Bangalore et al., 'β-Blocker Use and Clinical Outcomes in Stable Outpatients With and Without Coronary Artery Disease', *Journal of the American Medical Association*, 2012; 308 (13): 1340–1349.

257 **He subsequently carried out a similar exercise ...** Sripal Bangalore et al., 'Renin angiotensin system inhibitors for patients with stable coronary artery disease without heart failure: systematic review and meta-analysis of randomized trials', *British Medical Journal*, 2017; 356: j4.

259 **These reduce the risk ...** Ioanna Koniari et al., 'Pharmacologic prophylaxis for atrial fibrillation following cardiac surgery: a systematic review', *Journal of Cardiothoracic Surgery*, 2010, 5:121; Steven J. Kernis et al., 'Does Beta-Blocker Therapy Improve Clinical Outcomes of Acute Myocardial Infarction After Successful Primary Angioplasty?', *Journal of the American College of Cardiology*, 2004; 43: 1773–9.

260 **As for the longer term ...** Karen Okrainec et al., 'Cardiac Medical Therapy in Patients After Undergoing Coronary Artery Bypass Graft Surgery', *Journal of the American College of Cardiology*, 2005; 45: 177–84.

260 **They confer no benefit ...** Apurva A. Motivala et al., 'Predictors, Trends, and Outcomes (Among Older Patients ≥65 Years of Age) Associated With Beta-Blocker Use in Patients With Stable Angina Undergoing Elective Percutaneous Coronary Intervention', *Journal of the American College of Cardiology: Cardiovascular Interventions*, 2016, Vol. 9, DOI:10.1016/j.jcin.2016.05.048.

260 **There is now general agreement that** ... Dimitri Kalavrouziotis et al., 'Should all patients be treated with an angiotensin-converting enzyme inhibitor after coronary artery bypass graft surgery? The impact of angiotensin-converting enzyme inhibitors, statins, and β-blockers after coronary artery bypass graft surgery', *American Heart Journal*, 2011; 162: 836–43.

260 **Here the two relevant studies show** ... Genell L. Knatterud et al., 'Long-Term Effects on Clinical Outcomes of Aggressive Lowering of Low-Density Lipoprotein Cholesterol Levels and Low-Dose Anticoagulation in the Post Coronary Artery Bypass Graft Trial', *Circulation: Journal of the American Heart Association*, 11 July 2000, Vol. 102(2), pp. 157–165.

260 **Following coronary angioplasty** ... Grish R. Mood et al., Meta-Analysis of the Role of Statin Therapy in Reducing myocardial Infarction Following Elective Percutaneous Coronary Intervention', *American Journal of Cardiology*, 2007; 100: 919–923.

Figures and Tables Credits

Figure 1.1: Information derived from 'Compendium of Health Statistics', Office of Health Economics, 2009 and 'Prescriptions Dispensed in the Community England 2003–13', Health & Social Care Information Centre, 2014.

Table 1.1: Information derived from *Deadly Medicines and Organised Crime*, Peter C. Gotzsche, Radcliffe Publishing, 2013.

Figure 1.2: 'The Rise and Fall of Ischaemic Heart Disease, Reuel Stallones, *Scientific American*, Vol. 243, pp. 43–9, 1980. Reproduced with permission. Copyright © 1980 Scientific American, a division of Nature America, Inc. All rights reserved.

Table 1.2: Information derived from 'Reduction in Incidence of Coronary Heart Disease', Lipid Research Clinics Coronary Primary Prevention Trial, *Journal of the American Medical Association*, 1984, Vol. 251, pp. 351–73.

Table 2.1: Veterans' Administration Co-operative Study Group, 'Effects of Treatment on Morbidity in Hypertension', *Journal of the American Medical Association*, 1967, Vol. 202, pp. 1028–33. Presentation of data from Gilbert Welch, *Overdiagnosed*, Beacon Press, 2011.

Figure 2.1: Information derived from 'Hypertension Detection and Follow-up Program Collective Group: A Progress Report', *Circulation Research*, 40 (Suppl. 1), 106–109, 1977.

Table 2.2: Information derived from Medical Research Council, 'Medical Research Council Trial of Mild Hypertension: Principal Results', *British Medical Journal*, 1985, Vol. 291, pp. 97–103.

Figure 2.2: Information based on Figure 2.1 derived from 'Hypertension Detection and Follow-up Program Collective Group: A Progress Report', *Circulation Research*, 40 (Suppl. 1), 106–109, 1977.

Table 2.3: Information derived from 'Common and less common adverse effects of antihypertensives', Y. Trinder, *South African Family Practice Journal*, 2012, Vol. 54 (2), (Suppl. 1), pp. S31–S32.

Figure 3.1: Information derived from 'Coronary Heart Disease in Seven Countries', Ancel Keys, 'XVII. The Diet', *Circulation*, Vol. 41, (Suppl. 1), pp. 1–211, 1 April 1970. Reproduced by kind permission of Wolter Kluwer Health, Inc.

Figure 3.2: *Eat Your Heart Out*, James Le Fanu, MacMillan, 1987.

Figure 3.3: *Eat Your Heart Out*, James Le Fanu, MacMillan, 1987.

Figure 3.4: *The Rise and Fall of Modern Medicine*, James Le Fanu, Abacus, 2011.

Table 3.1: Information derived from 'Reduction in Incidence of Coronary Heart Disease', Lipid Research Clinics Coronary Primary Prevention Trial, *Journal of the American Medical Association*, 1984, Vol. 251, pp. 351–73.

Table 3.2: Information derived from 'Reduction in Incidence of Coronary Heart Disease', Lipid Research Clinics Coronary Primary Prevention Trial, *Journal of the American Medical Association*, 1984, Vol. 251, pp. 351–73.

Table 4.1: *The Rise and Fall of Modern Medicine*, James Le Fanu, Abacus, 2011.

Figure 4.1: Information derived from *The Journal of Lipid Research*, 1998, 39, pp. 44–50.

Figure 4.2: Information derived from 'Changing Disease Definitions: Implications on Disease Prevalence', L. M. Schwartz and S. Woloshin, *Effective Clinical Practice*, 1999, Vol. 2, pp. 76–85. Reproduced with permission from Gilbert Welch, *Overdiagnosed*, Beacon Press, 2011.

Table 4.2: Information derived from 'Prevention of Coronary Heart Disease in Men with Hypercholesterolemia', J. Shepherd et al, for the West of Scotland Coronary Prevention Study Group, *New England Journal of Medicine*, Vol. 333, pp. 1301–1307, 1996, and 'Reducing the Risk of Coronary Events: Evidence from the Scandinavian Simvastatin Survival Study (4S)', J. Kjekshus, for the Scandinavian Simvastatin Survival Study Group, *American Journal of Cardiology*, Vol. 76, pp. 64–80, 1995.

Table 4.3: Information derived from 'Prevention of Coronary Heart Disease in Men with Hypercholesterolemia', J. Shepherd et al, for the West of Scotland Coronary Prevention Study Group, *New England Journal of Medicine*, Vol. 333, pp. 1301–1307, 1996, and 'Reducing the Risk of Coronary Events: Evidence from the Scandinavian Simvastatin Survival Study (4S)', J. Kjekshus, for the Scandinavian Simvastatin Survival Study Group, *American Journal of Cardiology*, Vol. 76, pp. 64–80, 1995.

Table 4.4: Information derived from 'Pravastatin in elderly individuals at risk of vascular disease (PROSPER): a randomised controlled trial', *The Lancet*, 2002, Vol. 360, pp. 1623–30.

Figure 4.3: Information derived from 'Deaths registered by cause, gender and age', England and Wales, Office for National Statistics, 2016 and 'Prescriptions Dispensed in the Community, England 2003–13', Health & Social Care Information Centre.

Figure 4.4: Information derived from graphic 'Good for the Heart?' from Michael Brooks, *Cholesterol Wars*, *New Scientist*, 11 February 2017, pp. 29–32 © 2017 New Scientist Ltd. All rights reserved. Distributed by Tribune Content Agency.

Figure 5.1: Reproduced from *British Medical Journal*, 'Maturity onset diabetes mellitus: response to intensive dietary management', D. R. Hadden, D. A. Montgomery, R. J. Skelly, E. R. Trimble, J. A. Weaver, E. A. Wilson, K. D. Buchanan, Vol. 3, pp. 276–78, 2 August 1975, with permission from British Medical Journal Publishing Group Ltd.

Table 6.1: Information derived from NHS website: Annex A:Quality Indicators-summary of points-NHS Digital.

Table 7.1: Information derived from Cynthia M. Boyd et al, 'Clinical Practice Guidelines and Quality of Care for Older Patients With Multiple Comorbid Diseases', *Journal of the American Medical Association*, August 10, 2005, Vol. 294, No.6, pp. 216–24.

Figure 7.1: Helen Colhoun and Patricia Prescott-Clarke, 'Health Survey for England 1994', HMSO, 1996. Crown Copyright. Queen copyright information is reproduced with the permission of the Controller of HMSO and the Queen's Printer for Scotland.

Table 8.1: Information derived from 'Mild hypertension in people at low risk', Professor Stephen Martin, *British Medical Journal*, 349, 2014, g5432; 'Should people at low risk of cardiovascular disease take a statin?', Dr John D. Abramson, *British Medical Journal*, 347, 2013, f6123; 'The low carbohydrate diet to achieve weight loss and improve HbA1c Type 2 diabetes', Dr David Unwin, *Practical Diabetes*, Vol. 31, 2014, pp. 1–4; Teppo L. N. Järvinen, *British Medical Journal*, 350, 2015, h2088; 'Long-term Use of Cardiovascular Drugs', Professor Desmond Julian, *Journal of the American College of Cardiology*, 66, 2015, pp. 1273–85.

Table A1.1: Information derived from 'Randomised Trial of Effect of Alendronate on Risk of Fracture in Women with Existing Vertebral Fractures', Dennis M. Black, *The Lancet*, 1996, Vol. 348, pp. 1535–41.

Table A1.2 Information derived from 'Effect of Alendronate on Risk of Fracture in Women With Low Bone Density but Without Vertebral Fractures', Steven R. Cummings, *Journal of the American Medical Association*, 1998, 280: 2077–2082.

Figure A1.1: Reproduced from *British Medical Journal*, 'Overdiagnosis of bone fragility in the quest to prevent hip fracture', Teppo L. N. Järvinen, Karl Michaëlsson, Jarkko Jokihaara, Gary S. Collins, Thomas L. Perry, Barbara Mintzes, Vijaya Musini, Juan Erviti, Javier Gorricho, James M. Wright, Harri Sievänen, Vol. 350, h2088, 26 May 2015, with permission from British Medical Journal Publishing Group Ltd.

Table A2.1: Information derived from 'A Randomized Trial of Propranolol in Patients With Acute Myocardial Infarction', *Journal of the American Medical Association*, March 26, 1982, Vol. 247 (12), pp. 1707–14.

Table A2.2: Information derived from 'Prevention of Cardiovascular Events and Death with Pravastatin in Patients with Coronary Heart Disease and a Broad Range of Initial Cholesterol Levels', LIPID Study Group, *New England Journal of Medicine*, 1998; 339: 1349–57.

Figure A2.1: 'The history of coronary reperfusion', Frans Van de Werf, *European Heart Journal*, 14 July 2014, Volume 35, Issue 37, pp. 2510–15, by permission of Oxford University Press.

Argentum Medical Illustrations Ltd is responsible for producing the original graphs or redrawing: Figures 2.1, 2.2, 3.1, 4.2, 4.3, 4.4, 5.1, 7.1 and A1.1.

Index

Index